Weapons of Mass Destruction, CBRN, and HAZMAT Incident Management

Mark D. Harris

MD, MPH, MBA, MDiv, PhD, ThM, DBAc

Colonel (retired), US Army

Firefighter and Chaplain, Beaver Volunteer Fire Department, WV

Chaplain, Southern Baptist Disaster Response

Cover design by Nancy Harris
Image used under license from Shutterstock.com

MD Harris Institute Publishing

Daniels, WV

eBook ISBN 978-1-7343617-9-7

Print ISBN 978-1-7343617-8-0

This book is dedicated to my
teammates at the Beaver Volunteer Fire Department,
to my colleagues in Dr. Stagger's Medical Director's Group,
to my brothers and sisters in Southern Baptist Disaster Relief, and
to the courageous men and women in emergency and disaster services
in West Virginia.

Table of Contents

Contents

Introduction

Our world has no end of dangers, and the same technology that ameliorates these dangers can be the technology that causes them. At least 39 countries, as well as terrorist and other hostile groups, possess weapons of mass destruction, including chemical, biological, radiological, and nuclear weapons. Modern industry uses over 350,000 different chemicals and mixtures of chemicals worldwide.[1] In the US, four billion tons of hazardous materials are shipped annually by highway, rail, water, or air.[2] Industries use these chemicals to make cars, power cell phones, produce food, and heal illness and injuries. But these same materials, used in wrong ways, at wrong times, or in wrong doses, can harm, kill, and destroy.

For centuries, chlorine has been used for bleaching textiles, for disinfection, to purify drinking water, and to slow the decay of animal products, like catgut used in violin strings. In its gaseous form, chlorine was the earliest chemical agent used in World War I. Likewise, the need for pesticides to kill lice and stop louse-borne typhoid in interwar Germany prompted the development of Zyklon B. Zyklon B was the nerve agent later responsible for the deaths of millions of Jews, Christians, and prisoners of war, in the Holocaust.[3]

Armies have used biological agents, or at least the threat of infection, against enemies for millennia. At the battle of Leignitz (1241), Tartars burned reeds which produced a foul-smelling smoke when the wind was blowing towards the Polish forces. Thinking that the smoke carried a deadly disease, the Polish forces broke and ran, and the Tartars massacred them.[4] The Greek and Roman armies of antiquity poisoned wells with carcasses, thereby denying their use to enemies. In 1346 at the Siege of Caffa, Tartars catapulted the bodies of plague victims into the city, contributing to the spread of the Black Death (Europe, Asia, Africa, bubonic plague, 1346-1353). The defending Genoese fled back to Italy, thus triggering the greatest disease outbreak in history.[5] During World War II, Unit 731 of the Imperial Japanese Army slaughtered hundreds of thousands of Chinese, Koreans, and prisoners of war while experimenting with biological and chemical agents.[6]

[1] Janet Pelley, "Number of Chemicals in Commerce Has Been Vastly Underestimated ," Acs.org (Chemical and Engineering News, American Chemical Society, February 12, 2020), https://cen.acs.org/policy/chemical-regulation/Number-chemicals-commerce-vastly-underestimated/98/i7.

[2] International Association of Fire Chiefs and National Fire Protection Association, *Fundamentals of Fire Fighter Skills and Hazardous Materials Response* (Burlington, Ma: Jones & Bartlett Learning, 2020), 1076.

[3] William L. Shirer, *The Rise and Fall of the Third Reich: A History of Nazi Germany* (1960; repr., New York: Simon & Schuster, 2011), 270,272.

[4] Harold T. Cheshire, "The Great Tartar Invasion of Europe," *The Slavonic Review* 5, no. 13 (1926): 89–105, https://www.jstor.org/stable/4202032. Contribution from Modern Humanities Research Association. Some historians interpret this action as a smokescreen to hide a feigned retreat for the Tartar cavalry.

[5] Mark Wheelis, "Biological Warfare at the 1346 Siege of Caffa," *Emerging Infectious Diseases* 8, no. 9 (September 2002): 971–75, https://doi.org/10.3201/eid0809.010536.

[6] Sheldon H Harris, *Factories of Death: Japanese Biological Warfare 1932-45 and the American Cover-Up.* (New York: Routledge, 2015).

People have died from cancer induced by environmental and solar radiation since pre-history, though they did not know the cause. It has only been since Henry Becquerel discovered radiation in 1896, though, that man has known what caused or contributed to many such unexplained deaths. Radiation in war, such as Hiroshima and Nagasaki, killed over 200,000 people. Radiation accidents have most likely killed under 2,000. Such accidents, like the one in Goiânia, Brazil in 1987, still occur.

Authorities have been warning medical and emergency services personnel and organizations to be prepared for CBRN incidents, both intentional and unintentional, for decades. It may feel, to some, like an overblown threat. But it is not. This book describes many historical events and CBRN exposures, but there are undoubtedly others which went unrecognized. Despite the recent elimination of the US chemical weapon inventory, threats from toxic chemicals have only grown. As more nations get "the bomb," nuclear dangers grow. Finally, as lab and processing equipment improves, biological agents become easier to acquire and use.

All emergency and disaster responders should be familiar with WMD/CBRN hazards. Disaster response organizations such as the Southern Baptist Disaster Relief (SBDR), Samaritan's Purse, the Salvation Army, World Vision, and the American (or International) Red Cross (or Crescent) clean out areas damaged by flood, fire, wind, or earthquake that may be contaminated with toxic materials. Terrorists may target disaster relief operations to kill responders, hamper operations, and garner more publicity.

Many WMD/CBRN management guides focus on specific organizations, such as the military, or on specific groups, like physicians. Fire service personnel, other than HAZMAT specialists, have limited training and equipment to recognize and manage WMD/CBRN incidents. For example, firefighters cover basic HAZMAT in Firefighter 1 but often get no more training in WMD/CBRN during their time in the Fire Service. In some departments, fire apparatus' have zero or one radiation detectors. And yet, fire personnel will often be the first to respond to a WMD/CBRN incident.

A WMD/CBRN incident can be more than a terrorist or war attack. Hazardous material (HAZMAT) accidents abound. Toxic Industrial Chemicals (TICs) such as chlorine, phosgene, cyanide, and even organophosphates are more commonly found in factories than in terrorist camps. Biological agents such as anthrax can cause disease from spores that exist naturally in soil. The US has several cases of plague, tularemia, and hemorrhagic fevers each year from natural exposure. One flooded basement that I cleaned out with my SBDR team in July 2023 was heavily contaminated with rat feces, a set up for inhaled hantavirus pulmonary system, which kills up to 1/3 of people infected.[7]

Doctors in primary care clinics and hospitals may be the first to diagnose biological exposures or attacks. First responders have the opportunity to assess the entire incident scene, so they

---

[7] CDC, "Signs & Symptoms," Centers for Disease Control and Prevention, 2018, https://www.cdc.gov/hantavirus/hps/symptoms.html.

should learn to diagnose chemical and radiation incidents, and make a preliminary diagnosis of biological events. The following information is critical to making good diagnoses:

1. Characteristics of agent – gas, liquid, solid, odor, color, amount, lighter or heavier than air.
2. Scene – leaking tanks, machinery, other containers for the agent, other casualties, coworkers who may know the victim, or something about the dangers, uninvolved witnesses. Rodents or evidence of their presence such as feces. Dead animals, plants, or people.
3. Information - what happens routinely at this location, Safety Data Sheet (SDS), any previous problems.
4. Other factors such as temperature, wind, or humidity which may impact the release of chemicals or radiation or spread anthrax or botulinum spores.
5. Other injuries or illnesses.
6. Need for law enforcement if it is considered a crime scene or terrorist incident.

Secondary and tertiary health care providers will have a fraction of the above information. The little that they have will have been reported by someone else. Since the first responder has far more information, he or she must figure out what is going on and deal with it effectively.

Hazardous chemicals include those used in manufacturing, transportation, healthcare, and other fields. *Hazardous waste* includes chemicals and other substances created by or contaminated during commercial processes (i.e., manufacturing, health care, research, and development). Such waste is of no further use to the producer. Rags soaked in toxic chemicals, dirty needles from clinics, non-functional equipment, and blood-soaked bandages are examples of hazardous waste. Hazardous chemicals are needed for future processes, but hazardous waste is discarded.

Companies may not use the same care to dispose of waste as they do to save chemicals and other materials that they can still profit from. Also, hazardous chemicals are usually in their pure form, while hazardous waste is often a mix of chemicals, cleaning materials, and other substances. In a chemical mix, especially because waste chemicals can react with each other, it can be hard to tell what dangers lurk. First responders, disaster recovery personnel, and tertiary medical personnel must consider how to protect and treat themselves and others in this complicated environment.

Years ago, I was serving as a medical officer in the US Army. A patient presented to our emergency room with difficulty breathing. Terrorist attacks had heightened concern about mailroom safety, and this patient was a postal worker. Another postal worker came in a little later with similar complaints. We informed our higher commands, both medical and line, and cared for the patients while they began investigating. After a few hours, we learned the outcome. Worrying about terrorism, the postal workers thought that if one cleaner, bleach, was good, then two cleaners, bleach and ammonia, must be better. So they, and two others in the mailroom, mixed bleach and ammonia, generating chloramine gas.[8] Two people remained asymptomatic, and the two in our emergency room with chloramine pneumonitis, gradually improved and were sent home. As subject matter experts, we helped develop an instructional course on mixing cleaners. The talk was given to mailroom personnel in the region.

Another name used to refer to CBRN incidents is Weapons of Mass Destruction (WMD) incidents. According to US Code Title 18, Part 1, Chapter 113b, 2332a, a WMD is:

> Any destructive device, such as an explosive, incendiary, or poison gas bomb, grenade, rocket having a propellant charge of more than 4 oz (113 grams), missile having an explosive or incendiary charge of more than 0.25 oz (7 grams), mine, or similar device; (2) any weapon involving toxic or poisonous chemicals; (3) any weapon involving a disease organism; or (4) any weapon that is designed to release radiation or radioactivity at a level dangerous to human life.

Intent separates an accident from a terrorist incident, or at least a crime. Airplanes are critical to transportation in the US, and plane crashes are horrible tragedies. But to intentionally crash large passenger planes into the World Trade Center and the Pentagon is a heinous crime (US, 2001). Trains carry the goods that we depend on to survive in the modern world. Sometimes they derail, causing great damage. But intentionally bombing and derailing trains, such as occurred in Madrid in 2004, killing 193 people, deserves the harshest penalty.

Incidents involving CBRN/WMD involve many stakeholders. Local responders will quickly be joined by regional, state, and national personnel. The FBI will be at suspected crime scenes and the DOT will be at car or train wrecks. If it flies, or used to fly, the FAA will soon follow. OSHA and the EPA will appear, as well as an alphabet soup of others. Control and jurisdictional issues abound. Responders should know and follow the National Incident Management System (NIMS). In large events, disaster response groups will show up a little later to help put things back together.

This book summarizes WMD/CBRN management, including risks, agents, treatment, and decontamination. I have used the acronym CBRN instead of CBRNE because my focus is on parts 2, 3, and 4 of the WMD definition. Management of purely explosive injuries is well discussed in other documents. This work integrates guidance from fire fighter-, other first responder-, disaster relief worker-, and physician-facing resources to assemble what I believe is a unique book for WMD/CBRN issues. This book grew out of a lecture that I gave to a group of first responders at a meeting in Raleigh County WV on 13 July 2023. It is a summary of WMD/CBRN issues and does not replace usual training for firefighters, medical personnel, or other responders. Persons interested in such training should consult their firefighter, medical, and other instructional materials (such as those listed in the footnotes).

---

[8] This was similar to the chlorine gas used by both sides in World War I. They postal workers had created and experienced an accidental WMD.

The WMD/CBRN information presented below is basic, easily accessible, and easily understandable. The brevity and table format should make it useful for education and operations. Because of the overlap of WMD/CBRN with HAZMAT, HAZMAT notes are included when applicable.

Chapter I

First on Scene – Size Up and Incident Action Plan

The first task in any incident, WMD/CBRN/HAZMAT, car crash, structure fire, or anything else, is to find out what is going on (**Size Up**). This must be done safely to minimize the risk to others. While terrorists and enemies will not likely include a Safety Data Sheet (SDS) to let those they attack know which substances they are dealing with, toxic substance exposures associated with accidents usually come with information to help responders. SDSs, hazard identification (NFPA, military, OSHA), and shipping documents (including bills of lading, waybills, dangerous cargo manifests, and air bills) provide critical information to responders.

Size Up includes separating hazards from people. In a WMD/CBRN/HAZMAT incident, leaders establish hot, warm, and cold zones. The last part of Size Up is to inform command and notify all necessary responders. Eventually, someone must contact other stakeholders. Informing relevant parties includes letting them know what is happening, but also what on-scene leaders plan to do about it.

Scene Size Up

On arrival at a scene, the first task is to determine what is going on. Is it a common structure fire, a HAZMAT scene at a warehouse, or a terrorist attack from a dirty bomb contaminated with radium 226? Did a train derailment leak 20,000 gallons of kerosene into a hospital parking lot, or does the local emergency department have eight people who ate last night at the same restaurant and who are now complaining of abdominal pain and diarrhea? Fire departments respond to all hazards, not just fires and car wrecks. Emergency departments handle a huge variety of problems. The complexity and scope of emergency response is nothing like ever before.

The first part of size up is to be **safe** while sizing up the situation. Stay uphill and upwind from the incident if possible. Approach slowly, looking for markers (such as placards) just as you would look for flames and smoke when approaching a structure fire. Use binoculars to read the placards (when available) from a distance. Do a 360 degree walk around the scene and keep non-responders (like the public and the media) out while doing it. Talk to others at the scene to ascertain what happened. If you suspect a toxic substance is involved, try to identify it. Ensure that everyone is as safe as possible. Don the appropriate personal protective equipment (PPE) if you haven't already.

Try to identify the extent of the hazard. For example, if a leaking MC-307/DOT-407 tanker has a maximum capacity of 7,000 gallons, the bill of lading says that 7,000 gallons were loaded on to the tanker, and an estimated 6,000 gallons remain in the vehicle, the spill size is around 1,000 gallons.[9] Size can also be estimated by the area covered by a spill, such as a pool that is 10, 20, or 30 feet in diameter. Information on the concentration of the agent should be found on the shipping documents.

Safety data sheets (SDS) indicate the name of the substance, telephone numbers for contact personnel, hazards (including 1 through 4 level of severity), pictograms, routes of entry, exposure limits, precautionary statements, emergency procedures, and waste disposal. Notice that some chemical warfare agents, such as hydrogen cyanide and phosgene, are on the list of toxic industrial chemicals (TICs).

The National Fire Protection Association (NFPA) 704 Marking System is used for fixed facilities. OSHA uses the Hazardous Material Information System which is similar to the NFPA. DOT's Emergency Response Guidebook (ERG) provides first responders with information and instructions for transportation related HAZMAT incidents. Similar techniques will be used for other chemical CBRN agents.

The marking system of the Department of Transportation (DOT) includes environmental hazards, inhalation hazards, elevated temperature, and consumer commodity. The DOT system is only used for transporting materials.

The second part of size up is to **isolate**. In a WMD/CBRN/HAZMAT incident, establish hot, warm, and cold zones. Victims in the hot zone can be evacuated (with proper precautions including decontamination) or shelter in place (until further help arrives). As responders arrive, set up a command post and determine a basic incident plan.

The third part of size up is to **notify** the appropriate stakeholders about the nature of the incident, including the estimated number of casualties. Notification may include law enforcement, emergency medical services, dispatch, or someone else. Department and local standard operating procedures (SOPs) will dictate who notifies whom. Contact local medical facilities so they can prepare to receive casualties. If you have identified the agent involved, tell them. Teams responding to the incident can report to their chain of command, including the incident commander, using the CAN framework.[10]

1. Conditions – What is the current status of your team and what is happening regarding the incident from your perspective?
2. Actions – What have you and your team done since your last report, and what are you doing next?
3. Needs – What resources do you need to continue your work?

Size up answers the questions of what happened, what is likely to happen next, and what must we do about it? "What to do" is contained in the incident action plan.

---

[9] International Association of Fire Chiefs and National Fire Protection Association, *Fundamentals of Fire Fighter Skills and Hazardous Materials Response* (Burlington, MA: Jones & Bartlett Learning, 2020), 1171.
[10] International Association of Fire Chiefs and National Fire Protection Association, *Fundamentals of Fire Fighter Skills and Hazardous Materials Response* (Burlington, MA: Jones & Bartlett Learning, 2020), 1197.

Incident Action Plan

After size-up, the incident commander must determine an incident action plan (IAP).[11] The plan must include offensive actions, defensive actions, and sometimes non-intervention. Often leaders implement defensive operations first, confining a hazard. Once the hazard is confined, they move to offensive operations, which involve containing and ultimately eliminating the hazard. Such a plan is similar to a transitional fire attack, starting defensive and finishing offensive, done in routine structural firefighting. Non-intervention is also present in day-to-day firefighting, such as when an incident commander (IC) lets a small trash dump fire burn itself out.

1. Offensive actions – These are actions to directly mitigate the problem, typically within the hot zone. For example, a plan to stop hazardous material from leaking out of or otherwise escaping its container by plugging the hole would be an offensive action called containment.
2. Defensive actions – These are actions to hinder the spread or extension of the problem. For example, digging a trench to protect a waterway from a hazardous spill is a defensive action called confinement.
3. Non-intervention – Some events are self-limited, such as when a propane tank with a broken nozzle but not aflame empties itself into the atmosphere. Such a situation in a highly populated urban area may call for an offensive attack. The same scenario in a rural area with no one close enough to become a casualty might be handled with non-intervention. Other situations have such high risks and such low rewards that it is foolish to risk rescuers.

The sections of the IAP include:

1. Specific objectives
2. Clear work assignments for each responder
3. Resources needed to respond, including where and how to get them.
4. Organizational chart listing leadership people and positions.
5. Communication methods and channels
6. Medical plan – including emergency treatment, evacuation, and receiving facilities.
7. Site safety plan – This must consider law enforcement, as WMD/CBRN incident perpetrators sometimes stage secondary attacks. The plan should also include heat, cold, and other environmental contingencies.

The IAP guides the actions of all actors in an emergency site, from structure fire to HAZMAT to WMD. Size up is updated continuously with changing circumstances. The IAP is updated continually with new information from the Size-Up and with changes in leadership.

---

[11] International Association of Fire Chiefs and National Fire Protection Association, *Fundamentals of Fire Fighter Skills and Hazardous Materials Response* (Burlington, MA: Jones & Bartlett Learning, 2020), 1174.

Many WMD/CBRN/HAZMAT incidents will occur over large areas with significant populations of people who are not casualties of the agent. Part of the IAP must address what to do with those people. Should they be evacuated? If so, where will they go, and how will they get there? What needs will they have along the way, and once they arrive at their destination? Who will meet those needs? Should they shelter in place? If so, do they have the support they need to survive? This includes power, water, food, and medical care as needed. Should they be told to stay indoors? In such an incident, the IC is responsible for these decisions, and for these people. What about people who are missing? Should respondents mobilize search and rescue teams to find them, or is the danger too great?

For example, an intentional derailment of a train carrying a cyanide containing liquid may cause agent to leak into the parking lot of a nursing home. What should rescuers do? Tell the residents to shelter in place? Evacuate them? If so, how, when, and to where? At these moments, the IC feels the burden of leadership, because he or she makes decisions that will save, or cost, lives.

Table 1 - NFPA Hazard Identification[12]

Rating	Health (blue)	Flammability (red)	Instability (yellow)	Special (white)
4	Death or major injury w/ short exposure Examples: hydrogen cyanide, phosgene, diborane, methyl isocyanate, hydrofluoric acid	Rapidly vaporize in ambient conditions (< 25 C) Examples: gasoline, acetylene, propane, hydrogen gas, diborane	Can detonate on their own Examples: nitroglycerin, chlorine dioxide, nitrogen triiodide, manganese heptoxide, TNT, Picric acid	ACID – acid ALK – alkali COR – Corrosive OX – oxidizer W – reacts with water Radioactive
3	Serious temporary injury on short exposure Examples: liquid hydrogen, sulfuric acid, calcium hypochlorite, carbon monoxide, hexafluorosilicic acid, zinc chloride, sodium hydroxide	Can be ignited in ambient conditions (< 37 C), Liquids and solids (including finely divided suspended solids) that can be ignited under almost all ambient temperature conditions (e.g., acetone, ethanol).	Require a strong source to detonate Examples: ammonium nitrate, cesium, hydrogen peroxide	
2	Injury with intense exposure Examples: diethyl ether, ammonium phosphate, carbon dioxide, chloroform, DEET	< 93 C, Examples: diesel fuel, paper, sulfur and multiple finely divided suspended solids	Violent chemical reactions with water or high temperature and pressure Examples: white phosphorus, potassium, metallic sodium	
1	Minor injury Examples: acetone, sodium bromate, potassium chloride	> 93 C, Examples: mineral oil, ammonia, ethylene glycol	Normally stable except with high temperature and pressure Examples: propene, ammonium acetate, carbonic acid	
0	No injury, Examples: wood, sugar, salt, propylene glycol	Will not burn - Examples: carbon tetrachloride (CCl_4), silicon dioxide, perfluorohexane	Stable, Examples: helium, N2, carbon dioxide	

[12] International Association of Fire Chiefs and National Fire Protection Association, *Fundamentals of Fire Fighter Skills and Hazardous Materials Response* (Burlington, MA: Jones & Bartlett Learning, 2020), 1087.

Table 2 itemizes shipping documents to locate and review during size up for transportation accidents.

Table 2 – Shipping Documents for Hazardous Materials

Transport type	Name	Location	Other
Road	Bill of Lading, Freight Bill	Vehicle cab	
Rail	Waybill		A consist or train list specifies the contents of every car on the train
Water	Dangerous cargo manifest	Wheelhouse	Tube-like container
Air	Air bill	Cockpit	

Table 3 explains the Emergency Response Guidebook (ERG).

Table 3 – Summary of the Emergency Response Guidebook

ERG Section	Information Contained
Yellow	4,000 chemicals listed by UN/ID number. Includes emergency action guide number
Blue	4,000 chemicals listed alphabetically by name.
Orange	Organized by guide number, includes general hazard class, fire/explosion hazard, health hazards, and basic emergency actions. Guidance on protective clothing, evacuation, fire and spill included.
Green	Listed by UN/ID number, includes initial isolation distances, recommended size and shape of protective action zones, and toxic inhalation hazards. Chemicals listed in the Green section are extremely hazardous.

The ERG 2020 includes chemical agents (such as soman) and radiological sources (such as thorium). An ERG app is available for free download. The ERG is a must for WMD/CBRN initial response.

Firefighting Notes with WMD/CBRN/HAZMAT incidents

CBRN incidents pose specific challenges when they are present in a fire situation, such as might be the case in a dirty bomb or nuclear detonation. Also, some CBRN agents such as nerve agents and vesicants can burn if ignited.

1. Structural firefighting PPE (turnout gear) cannot protect a firefighter against chemicals like an agent-specific suit and respirator can.
2. Class A foam is useful for extinguishing ordinary fires but is not optimal for fires which include a CBRN component. Other foam classes are better, such as aqueous, alcohol resistant, fluoroprotein, or protein for burning liquids.
3. Turnout gear cannot stop gamma rays and neutrons, so employ time, distance, and shielding (TFS) strategies immediately. Radioactive sources must be dealt with effectively and quickly.

Container failure

In a classic WMD/CBRN incident, the perpetrator intended for the container to release its contents. A cylinder spewing cyanide gas may be intentionally opened, for example. Otherwise, responding personnel must ascertain why a container holding a toxic substance failed. In the Brazil case, the scrap dealer brought tragedy on himself by opening the case to get to the cesium.

1. Thermal failure – Heat or cold fractured the container.
2. Chemical failure – A chemical interaction within the container led to overpressure or disintegration, bursting the container.
3. Mechanical failure – Falling debris, shrapnel, or forklift forks punctured the container.

Time, Distance, and Shielding

The effects of radiological, and to some degree chemical, agents on people are influenced by the amount of time exposed, the distance from the source, and any protection a person may have (Time, Distance, and Shielding – TDS). Generally, a person exposed to radioactive material for one minute will get less radiation than someone exposed for five minutes. Likewise, a person ten meters away will get less radiation than a person one meter away. Finally, a person shielded by a rock wall or pile of dirt will get less exposure than a person without any such protection. Broadly speaking, the same is true of chemical agents and toxic industrial chemicals (TICs).

First responders and incident commanders should use the principles of TDS to protect themselves and incident victims. After the initial response, which was chaotic, the Soviets used time, distance, and shielding to protect Russians, Byelorussians, and Ukrainians from radiation sickness after the Chernobyl nuclear power plant disaster in 1986. First, they tried to limit the time of exposure for those responding to the crisis. Second, they evacuated civilians away from a 30 km ring around the plant. Third, they built a huge earthen tomb around and over the stricken reactor to provide shielding. The TDS principle is related to the idea of separating the people from the problem in any way possible.

Chapter 2

Categories and Characteristics of Chemical Agents and Common Toxic Industrial Chemicals

In prehistory, man encountered chemicals which were mostly natural. Over the millennia our ancestors developed technologies requiring chemicals to extract metal from ores, separating chemicals from plants to get dyes, medicines, and perfumes, and making pottery, glass, and glazes. Early chemistry made fat into soap and copper and tin into bronze.

Modern chemistry began in the early 1700s and introduced thousands, and later hundreds of thousands, of organic and inorganic chemicals. Chemistry has served mankind, examples of which include petroleum to move things and fertilizers to grow crops. Chemistry has also, however, made us more effective at destroying each other and the world around us.

Chemical Agents (exposure by intoxication)

1. Nerve (organophosphates) – GA (Tabun), GB (Sarin), GD (Soman), GF (Cyclosarin), VX, Russian agents in the Novichok class (i.e., A-232).
2. Blistering (vesicants) – mustard, Lewisite
3. Blood agents (cyanides)
4. Lung/pulmonary/choking agents (phosgene, chlorine)
5. Incapacitants (opioid and anticholinergic incapacitating agents)
6. Riot control
7. Pharmaceuticals (illicit and commercial drugs) – opioids (fentanyl), stimulants (cocaine), or legal drugs at supratherapeutic or toxic doses.

Chemical agents (or chemical warfare agents) may have usefulness outside killing, but their primary goal is to eliminate enemies.

A toxic industrial chemical (TIC) is defined as a chemical, excluding chemical warfare agents, that has an LCt50 (Lethal concentration for 50% of population exposed over a given time, t) less than 100,000 mg-min/m^3 in any mammalian species and are produced in quantities exceeding 30 tons annually at any one production facility.[13] Examples of TICs include Phosgene (CG), Hydrogen chloride (HCl), Ammonia (NH_3), Perfluoro-isobutylene (PFIB), Oxides of nitrogen (NOx), and White phosphorus smoke. Toxic industrial chemicals (TICs) may be used to destroy, but their primary goal is to facilitate some processes intended to make life better. In both cases, first responders react to spills, releases, and other problems to limit damage caused by these dangerous chemicals. Disaster relief personnel may encounter TICs in household basements, schools, churches, warehouses set up as shelters, and other unexpected locations.

[13] Gregory R Ciottone, *Disaster Medicine* (Philadelphia: Elsevier/Mosby, 2016), 471.

Table 4 - Common Toxic Industrial Chemicals (exposure by intoxication)[14]

Agent	Molecular Weight	Boiling Point	Freezing Point	Distinctive Odor	Compartment of Action	Concentrated Exposure Limits (ppm)
Phosgene (CG)	99	7.6°C	−128°C	Newly mown hay	Peripheral	0.1
Hydrogen chloride (HCl)	36.46	−85°C	−114°C	Pungent	Peripheral	5
Ammonia	17.03	−33.4°C	−77.7°C	Sharp, intensely irritating	Central	50
Perfluoro-isobutylene	Polymer	214°C −217°C	257°C −263°C	None	Peripheral	0.01
Oxides of nitrogen (NOx)	28.1	−196°C	−210°C	Irritating	Peripheral	25
White phosphorus smoke	123.895	280°C	44.1°C	Garlic-like		1

The presence of dead or dying animals, birds, insects, or plants in the area suggests a chemical incident. Terrorists may leave tell-tale items behind, like gloves, chemical suits, respirators, and containers that they used to protect themselves when they released the agent. Preparation materials like scales, thermometers, other lab equipment, and even chemistry books might be present at indoor releases. Look for dispersal items, such as trucks with mounted sprayers, hand or machine operated pumps, or even crop-dusting aircraft. Chemical releases are often indoors to kill the most people. If outdoors, they often happen on days with little wind since wind disperses the agent and decreases the effect. Additionally, perpetrators sometimes accidentally harm themselves. One of the victims that you find may be the terrorist.

The key is to notice items that appear out of place. Laboratories that produce drugs, for example, can readily be modified to produce explosives or chemical agents. Primary devices would account for the initial agent released. Secondary devices go off after primary devices and target first responders. The EVADE acronym is useful for finding secondary devices:[15]

---

[14] Daniel E. Banks, ed., *Medical Management of Chemical Casualties Handbook*, 5th ed. (Government Printing Office, 2014), https://medcoe.army.mil/borden-tb-med-mgmt-chemical-casualties.

[15] International Association of Fire Chiefs and National Fire Protection Association, *Fundamentals of Fire Fighter Skills and Hazardous Materials Response* (Burlington, MA: Jones & Bartlett Learning, 2020), 1161.

1. Evaluate the scene for areas in which secondary devices could be placed.
2. Visually scan operating areas for a secondary device before providing patient care.
3. Avoid touching or moving anything that could hide a secondary device.
4. Designate and enforce scene control zones.
5. Evacuate victims, other responders, and nonessential personnel as quickly and safely as possible.

On 20 March 1995, the Japanese doomsday cult Aum Shinrikyo released sarin gas in a Tokyo subway. Twelve people died and 5500 were injured.[16] Previously, the group had released clostridium botulinum toxin outside the Japanese parliament, hoping to kill as many legislators as possible.

Examples of Effects of Specific Chemicals

"[C]arfentanil is the perfect terrorist weapon," acting CIA director Michael J. Morel wrote. "It is readily available in large quantities. It comes in several forms—including tablets, powder, and spray. It can be absorbed through the skin or through inhalation. It acts quickly ... In short, a single terrorist attack using carfentanil could kill thousands of Americans."[17]

Pesticides are often organophosphate chemicals similar to nerve agents. Zyklon B is an infamous example. Another, more modern example, is malathion. Malathion is an organophosphate similar to chemical nerve agents that is used for outdoor insect control, treatment of head and body lice and scabies.[18] Malathion can be fatal if ingested, as in the following true account:

> A 4-year-old girl drank malathion, an organophosphate pesticide. She was brought to a clinic after developing vomiting and diarrhea. She was also minimally responsive and struggling to breathe due to excess lung secretions, all toxic effects of this type of pesticide. She was given several doses of atropine (a drug that may help reverse the toxic effects of organophosphates) as well as pralidoxime (an antidote that may also reverse toxic effects of organophosphates) at maximum dosages and admitted to the hospital.
>
> The child's symptoms worsened. Twelve hours after she presented, a breathing tube was inserted and she was placed on a ventilator. Her physicians continued to treat her

---

[16] Erica Simons, "Faith, Fanaticism, and Fear: Aum Shinrikyo--the Birth and Death of a Terrorist Organization | Office of Justice Programs," www.ojp.gov, 2006, https://www.ojp.gov/ncjrs/virtual-library/abstracts/faith-fanaticism-and-fear-aum-shinrikyo-birth-and-death-terrorist.

[17] Becky Little, "How Opioids Were Used as Weapons during the Moscow Theater Hostage Crisis," HISTORY, August 23, 2018, https://www.history.com/news/opioid-chemical-weapons-moscow-theater-hostage-crisis.Updated: May 16, 2023, Original: May 25, 2018. Carfentanil is used to anesthetize large animals including elephants and rhinoceroses.

[18] CDC-Centers for Disease Control and Prevention, "CDC - Lice - Head Lice - General Information - Malathion FAQs," www.cdc.gov, September 17, 2020, https://www.cdc.gov/parasites/lice/head/gen_info/faqs_malathion.html.

with high doses of atropine and pralidoxime but two days later the child developed pulmonary edema (fluid build-up in the lungs) and continued to require a ventilator to breathe, as well as vasopressors (drugs that raise blood pressure when it is too low).

One of the child's physicians consulted the medical toxicologist at Poison Control to discuss the child's care and to ask how long the atropine and pralidoxime should be continued. The medical toxicologist explained that malathion can stay in fatty tissue such as the brain for up to 14 days and that there are case reports of needing to use these antidotes for up to 30 days.

Six days after the child ingested the malathion she remained on a ventilator with possible sepsis or pneumonia but had improved to the point that both the atropine and pralidoxime were discontinued. Eight days after she presented for medical care, she continued to need a ventilator to breathe, though her chest x-ray was improving. She had, however, developed ischemia (inadequate blood supply) of her small bowel and required surgery. The child remained in the hospital more than 2 weeks after drinking the malathion.[19]

More than 1,000 products in the US contain malathion, so first responders and medical personnel probably encounter it more than they realize. And malathion is only one of many, many hazardous chemical compounds. Such toxic chemicals are closely related to chemical warfare agents and can be used for nefarious purposes just like chemical warfare agents.

---

[19] Rose Ann Gould Soloway, "Pesticide and Nerve Agents: Similar Poisons, Similar Symptoms," www.poison.org, accessed August 2, 2023, https://www.poison.org/articles/pesticide-and-nerve-agent-commonality.

Chapter 3

Categories and Characteristics of Biological and Radiological Agents

Biological and radiological agents are natural. Until the modern day, they have not been synthesized or modified in laboratories but rather used in their natural state.

Biological Agents

1. Live agents (exposure by infection) – bacteria, fungi, viruses.
2. Toxins (exposure by intoxication) – chemicals originating from biological sources.

Biological warfare was practiced long before anyone knew about radiation or modern chemistry. Solon of Athens poisoned wells used by his enemies in the city of Kirrha with hellebore (Lenten Rose) during the First Sacred War (595-585 BC).[20] Lenten Rose contains veratrine, cyclopamine, and jervine, toxins which induce heart and nervous system failure, and cause birth defects. Symptoms can be debilitating and include diarrhea, nausea, vomiting, and bradycardia. The Assyrian army contaminated the wells of their enemies with ergot, a fungus which grows on grains such as wheat and rye. Patients poisoned with ergot can present with dizziness, convulsions, and psychosis. Death was common.

Anthrax has been and remains a major threat agent. Germany provided anthrax to the Finnish in their war against Imperial Russian forces in 1916.[21] The Imperial Japanese Army Unit 731 in World War II, the most notorious perpetrator of biological warfare in modern times, murdered prisoners with anthrax. An accident involving anthrax at the Soviet bioweapons facility in Sverdlovsk in 1979 killed 68 people.[22] The most recent major example in the US is the anthrax mailings after the terror attack on 911. In this attack, 22 people were infected and five died.

Agent Categories

1. Category A – Organisms that pose a risk to national security because they can be easily disseminated or transmitted from person to person and result in high mortality.
2. Category B – Organisms that are moderately easy to disseminate and have moderate morbidity rates and low mortality rates. Brucellosis, Q Fever, Ricin, and Vibrio Cholera fall into this category.
3. Category C – Pathogens that could be engineered for mass dissemination and high morbidity or mortality.

---

[20] Gregory R Ciottone, *Disaster Medicine* (Philadelphia: Elsevier/Mosby, 2016), 697.
[21] Gregory R Ciottone, *Disaster Medicine* (Philadelphia: Elsevier/Mosby, 2016), 700.
[22] Gregory R Ciottone, *Disaster Medicine* (Philadelphia: Elsevier/Mosby, 2016), 700.

Table 5 - Infection control issues for Biological Agents in likely terrorist usage[23]

Disease	Incubation Period (days)	Person to person transmission	Infection control standards
Anthrax	2-43	No	Standard
Botulism	1-3	No	Standard
Pneumonic plague	1-6	Yes	Droplet
Smallpox	7-17	Yes	Contact and airborne
Tularemia	1-14	No	Standard
Viral hemorrhagic fevers	2-21	Yes	Contact and airborne
Viral brain infection	2-14	No	Standard
Q Fever	2-14	No	Standard
Brucellosis	5-60	No	Standard
Glanders	10-14	No	Standard

Infection control matters to clinic and hospital personnel, but it also matters to first responders and disaster relief workers. Firefighters, for example, may not routinely wear masks for 911 calls. If the call is for one or more victims with unexplained cough, they should wear masks. Transmission information and infection control recommendations help protect victims and responders.

Radiological Agents (exposure by irradiation)

1. Alpha – large subatomic particle which can be blocked by clothing or paper. Alpha particles are most likely to cause damage when inhaled or ingested. Polonium is a powerful alpha emitter, and the doses used to kill Alexander Litvinenko came from a Russian nuclear power plant.
2. Beta – small subatomic particle which can be blocked by hard, thin, substances such as an aluminum plate. Beta particles cause superficial burns which resemble thermal burns like those seen from a blast wave.
3. Gamma – high energy photons with no mass. These can penetrate thick lead or earth.
4. Neutron – high energy particles which are highly penetrating. Neutrons can cause 20 times more damage to tissues than gamma waves. Neutrons slow or stop when they combine with hydrogen-rich substances, such as plastics and water.

Radioactive waste is often cited as a source of materials that could be obtained and used by terrorists in a CBRN event. Low level waste (LLW), about 94% of the total hazardous waste in the US, comes from hospitals, factories, and nuclear plants. Examples of low-level waste include wiping rags, mops, medical tubes, and carcasses of laboratory animals used in radiological

[23] Gregory R Ciottone, *Disaster Medicine* (Philadelphia: Elsevier/Mosby, 2016), 483. Hantavirus pulmonary syndrome is a category A bioterror threat.

research. LLW has been subdivided into four classes to guide disposal. Intermediate level waste (ILW) comprises about 6% of the total and includes resins, chemical sludge, and metal nuclear fuel cladding. High level waste (HLW) accounts for less than 1% of waste but 95% of radioactivity. HLW includes mostly uranium with fission products and transuranic elements generated in the reactor core.

Radiation accidents are uncommon. From 1944 to 2000, only 30 Americans died in accidents involving radiation. From 1950 to 2000, 59 deaths occurred. Worldwide, more than 120 people perished from acute radiation exposure.[24]

Personnel responding to a potential radiological event can get a lot of useful information by knowing from whence the radiological source came. If it came directly from a nuclear powerplant, it is likely more dangerous than sources from hospitals or industry.

Figure 1 – Nuclear Power Plant Schematic[25]

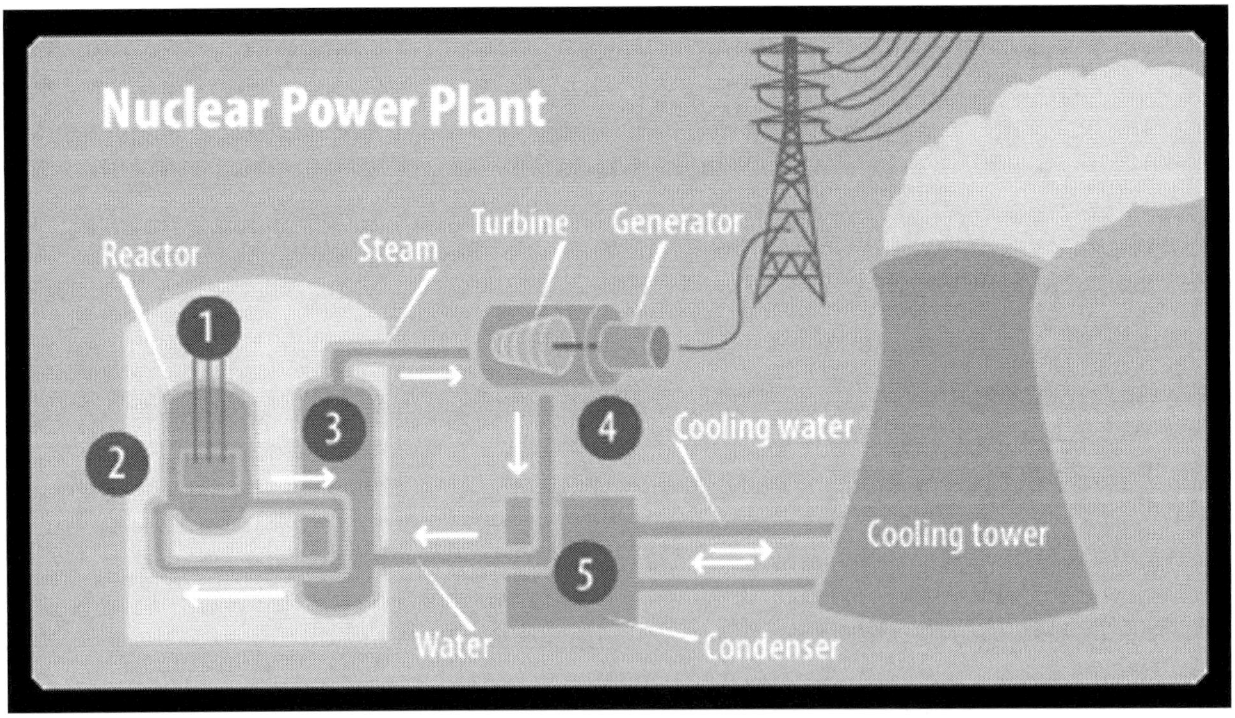

[24] Gregory R Ciottone, *Disaster Medicine* (Philadelphia: Elsevier/Mosby, 2016), 465.
[25] US EPA, OAR, Climate Change Division, "Nuclear Energy | a Student's Guide to Global Climate Change | US EPA," Epa.gov, May 9, 2017, https://archive.epa.gov/climatechange/kids/solutions/technologies/nuclear.html.

Figure 2 – Nuclear Power Plant Accident[26]

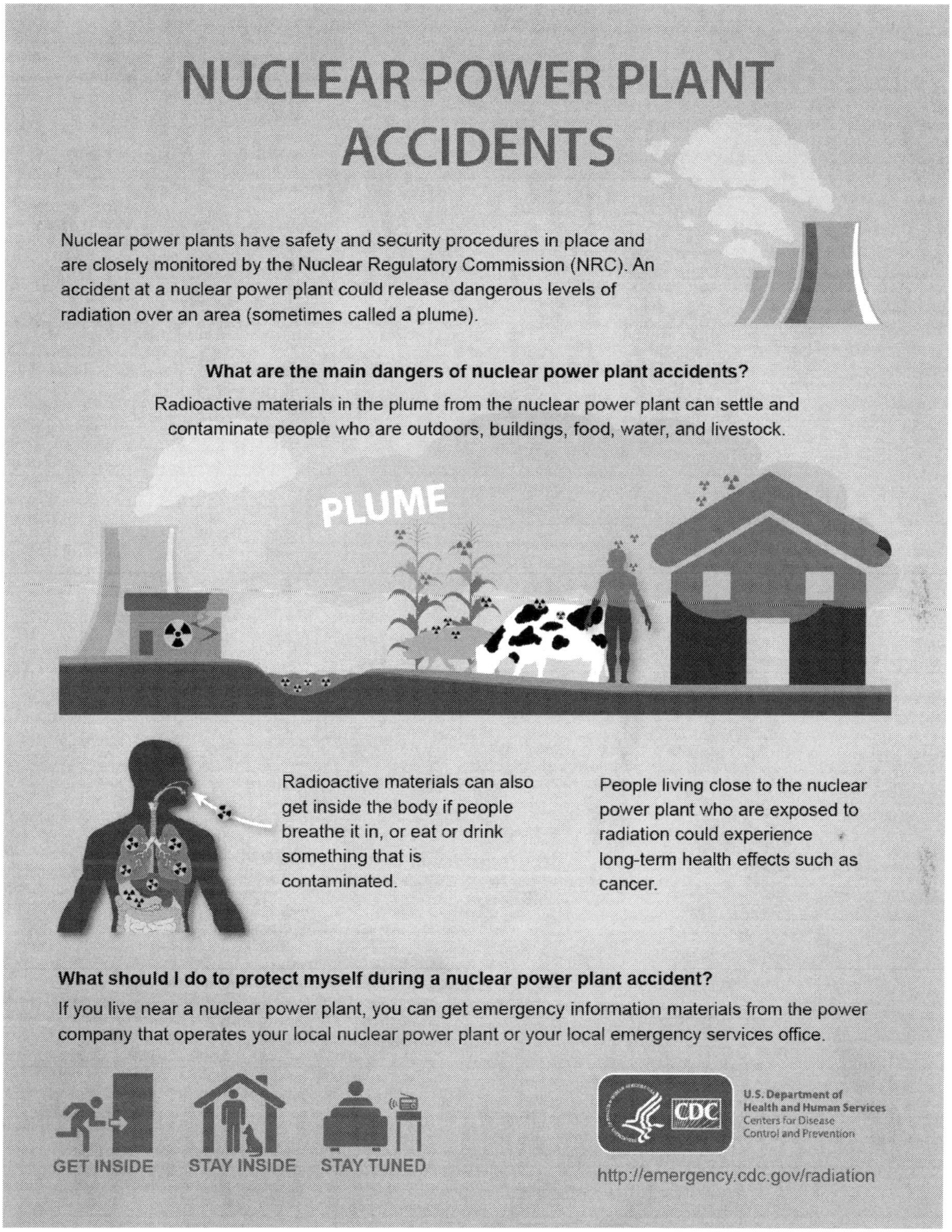

[26] Centers for Disease Control and Prevention, "Nuclear Power Plant Accidents | Chemicals, Radiation and Toxicology Infographics | NCEH," www.cdc.gov, February 6, 2020, https://www.cdc.gov/nceh/multimedia/infographics/nuclear_power_plant_accidents.html.

Figure 3 – Workplace Radiation Incidents[27]

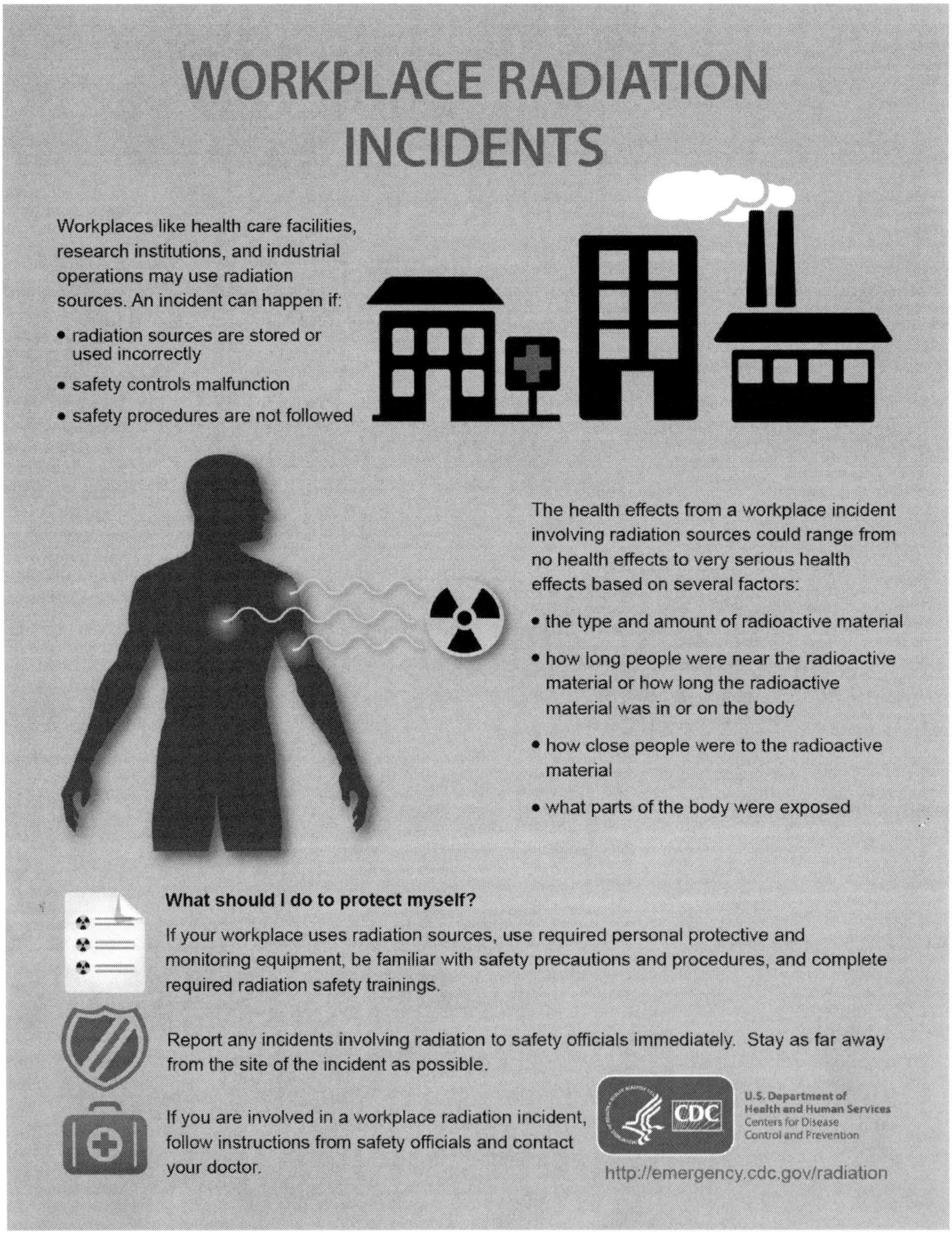

[27] Centers for Disease Control and Prevention, "Workplace Radiation Incidents | Chemicals, Radiation and Toxicology Infographics | NCEH," www.cdc.gov, January 23, 2023, https://www.cdc.gov/nceh/multimedia/infographics/workplace_radiation_incidents.html.

Figure 4 – Transportation Incidents[28]

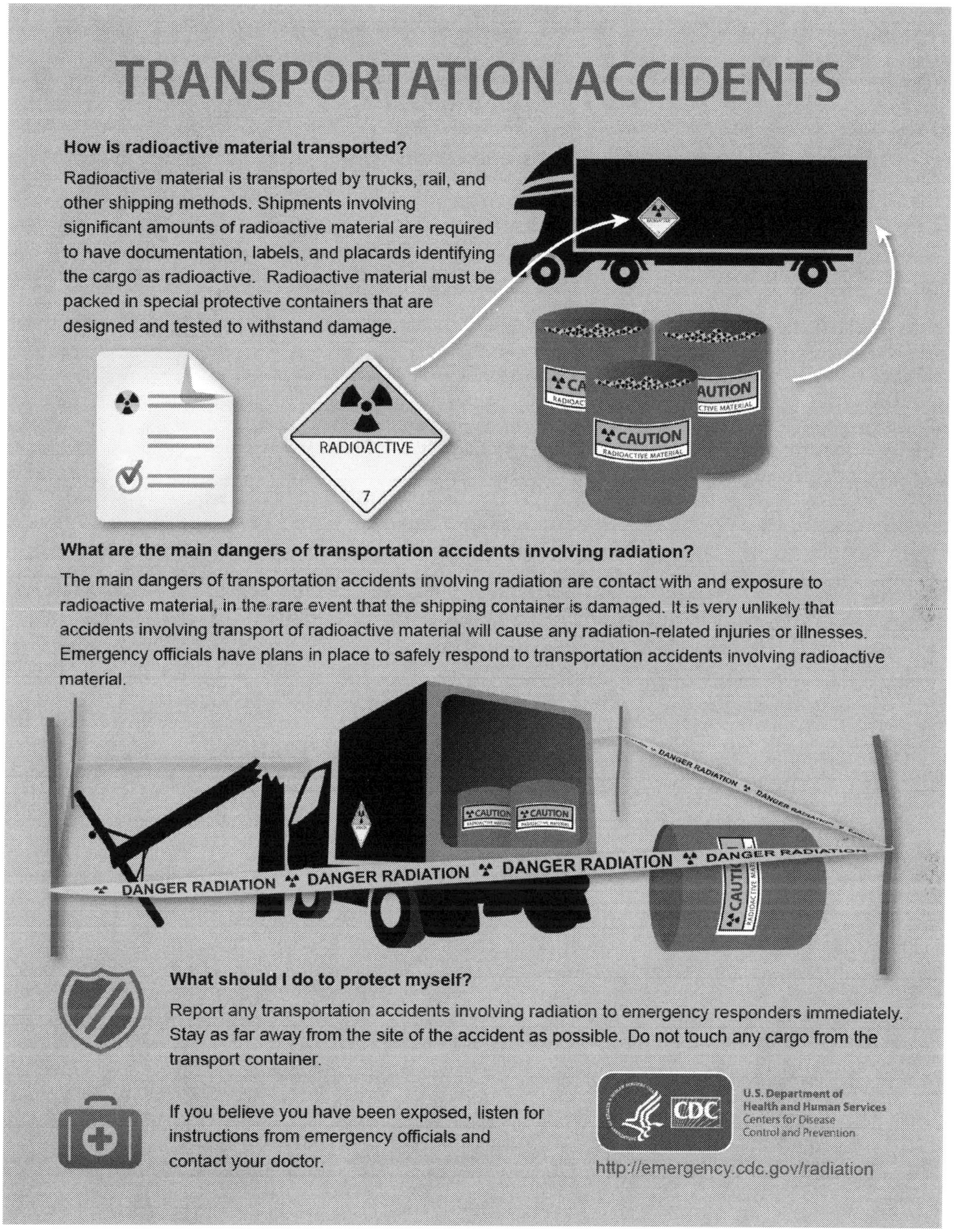

[28] Centers for Disease Control and Prevention, "Transportation Accidents | Chemicals, Radiation and Toxicology Infographics | NCEH," www.cdc.gov, January 23, 2023, https://www.cdc.gov/nceh/multimedia/infographics/transportation_accidents.html.

Chapter 4

WMD/CBRN General Principles

Despite the differences in WMD/CBRN and toxic industrial agents, they hold many commonalities. Chemicals, biological agents, and radiation share means of interacting with the human body. Chemicals, viruses, and radiological agents often change the deoxyribonucleic acid (DNA) which inhabits human cells. Due to the nature of the human body, exposures are the same for all WMD/CBRN agents – through the skin/mucous membranes or into an orifice.

Method of delivery – overt or covert

Secondary hazards

1. Contagious casualties – infected with pneumonic plague, smallpox, or some other contagious biological entity. Decontamination is not effective, so isolation is required to protect others from infection.
2. Contaminated casualties – people are primarily contaminated if they come directly into contact with an agent. They secondarily contaminate others if they pass the contamination on to them (people, equipment, supplies, facilities).
    a. External (absorption) – Contamination on the skin, mucous membranes, or clothing.
    b. Internal (inhalation or ingestion) – Contamination through the skin, in the respiratory tree, or in the gastrointestinal tract
    c. Wound (injection) – Contamination from damaging agent through skin protective layer. This represents a combined injury of conventional and radiological causes.

Direct contamination from a source is a primary hazard, while becoming contaminated from someone or something other than the primary source is a secondary hazard. For example, in the Goiânia accident in Brazil on 13 September 1987, thieves stole a teletherapy head containing cesium 137 source from an abandoned radiological hospital. They sold the head to a scrapyard owner, who broke open the capsule to see the glowing blue powder inside. Thinking it was a cosmetic, his six-year-old daughter spread the dust all over her skin. Other people inhaled or ingested the powder. Within days, the daughter and three others were dead. Two hundred fifty people were contaminated either directly from the powder in the capsule (primary contamination) or from the powder on someone's clothes or other objects (secondary contamination). Over 1,000 people suffered physical or emotional distress as a result.

Exposure Routes

1. Skin (percutaneous)
    a. Intact skin (transcutaneous) – Vesicants can damage the skin and cause systemic effects, while nerve agents, which are fat soluble) can directly penetrate intact skin.

i. Karen Wetterhahn (1948-1997), a chemist at Dartmouth, perished after dimethylmercury penetrated her gloved hand during an experiment.
ii. Sergei Skripal and his daughter Yulia were poisoned with a Russian nerve agent (A-234) from their doorknob and a perfume bottle (March 2018). Both survived.

b. Damaged skin – Intentional but small break in the skin to allow for admission of agent.
   i. Cleopatra (69-30 BC) died from intentionally provoking an asp to bite her (snake venom). The asp was the symbol of rule in Egypt.
   ii. Georgi Markov (1929-1978) was killed by Bulgarian agents when struck by a pellet of ricin hidden in the tip of an umbrella.
c. Wound – large disruption in skin integrity with contamination by CBRN agent(s).

2. Inhalation – This route provides the greatest risk for mass casualties. Masks, respirators, or SCBA gear protect against inhalation injury.
   a. Forty Chechen rebels took over the Dubrovka Theater on 23 October 2002, taking 850 hostages. After negotiations failed, on 26 October, Russians used carfentanil gas (opioid agent) against Chechen terrorists. All 40 rebels and 130 of 850 hostages died.
   b. Thirty to 60 workers die annually from inhalation of toxic industrial chemicals.[29]
3. Ingestion – The agent is taken into the body through the GI tract.
   a. Socrates (469 – 399 BC) died from ingesting hemlock.
   b. The Roman Emperor Claudius (10 BC – 54 AD) perished from ingesting belladonna (scopolamine, atropine).
   c. Arsenic in his medication may have contributed to the death of King George III (1738-1820) of Great Britain.
   d. Dr. Thomas Neil Cream (1850-1892) murdered at least eight people using strychnine before he was caught and executed.
   e. Alexander Litvinenko (1962-2006) was poisoned by polonium 210 placed in his tea on 1 Nov 2006.
   f. Alexei Navalny was poisoned by a Novichok nerve agent on 20 Aug 2020 but survived.
4. Eyes and mucous membranes – Significant local effects, such as pinpoint pupils from nerve agent or conjunctival irritation from mustard.

Physical Properties and Type of Release

1. Gas – Compressible, non-persistent agents which stay primarily in the air at ambient temperatures (chlorine).

---

[29] Bureau of Labor Statstics, U.S. Department of Labor, *The Economics Daily*, "Fatal Chemical Inhalations in the Workplace up in 2017," *Bls.gov*, October 24, 2019, https://www.bls.gov/opub/ted/2019/fatal-chemical-inhalations-in-the-workplace-up-in-2017.htm.

2. Vapor – Non-persistent agents which evaporate but stay mostly as a liquid at room temperature (nerve).
3. Liquid – Non-compressible persistent agents which are liquids at ambient temperature (i.e., mustard, nerve).
4. Aerosol – Liquids or solids which can be aerosolized and dangerous as particles in air (i.e., anthrax spores).
5. Solid – Non-compressible, fixed shape, and persistent (i.e., metallic sodium).
6. Ionizing radiation – radioactive material can be in any physical form.

Responders must consider both the agent and the characteristics of its release to predict outcomes. Mustard is a liquid, not a gas, at ambient temperatures, and so was dispersed to the trenches in World War I as a fine mist. Heavier than air, mustard settled into the lowest parts of trenches. In cool weather, it resumed its liquid form. Men stepping in pools of mustard suffered terrible chemical burns to their skin. Mustard is toxic but generally debilitating, not fatal. It persisted for a long time and was thus used to deny the use of an area by an enemy force. In World War I, for example, neither side could use trenches that had mustard agent pooled in the bottom.

Toxic industrial chemicals, and even non-toxic chemicals, invite the same consideration. Carbon dioxide (CO_2) and propane (C_3H_8) are heavier than air and so sink. They both displace atmospheric oxygen in trench and confined space situations. Without oxygen, anyone without SCBA or supplied air in those spaces will quickly lose consciousness. If not rescued, they will perish. But carbon dioxide is odorless, colorless, and tasteless, so responders do not realize they are entering a deadly environment.

Methane gas (CH_4) is lighter than air and will rise. Unless in a confined space, methane will not displace oxygen, but since it is flammable, methane may explode.

Commonly used gases that are lighter than air include hydrogen (H), helium (He), hydrogen cyanide (HCN), hydrogen fluoride (HF), methane (CH_4), ethylene (C_2H_4), diborane (B_2H_6), illuminating gas (methane/ethane), carbon monoxide (CO), ammonia (NH_3), neon (Ne), nitrogen (N2), and acetylene (C_2H_2). Most other commonly used gases are heavier than air and will fall to the lowest level available in an area.

The specific gravity (SG) of water (H_20) is 1.0, the SG of most fuels (gasoline, diesel fuel, motor oil, benzene) is less than 1.0, so these fuels float on water. The SG of carbon disulfide (CS_2), by contrast, 2.6, so water floats on top of CS_2.

The timing of symptoms provides an important clue about what type of CBRN attack is occurring and what specific agent is involved.

Effect Severity

1. Death – Lethal dose 50 (LD_{50}) by route of exposure (chemical or biological agents) or by duration of exposure (radiation). Lethal concentration time 50 (LCT_{50}) is used for inhalational exposures since concentration and duration of exposure can be inversely proportional to cause the same effect (death). Restated, a higher concentration of inhaled agent can cause death in a shorter time, and a lower concentration can cause death over a longer time.
2. Damage – Agent effects do not kill but require extensive medical resources (mustard agents) and/or leave permanent effects.
3. Incapacitating
4. Iatrogenic – medical countermeasures such as atropine have significant side effects (like tachycardia).
5. Psychological

Chapter 5

Casualty Assessment for WMD/CBRN

It bears repeating that field personnel, such as firefighters and paramedics, have the greatest opportunity to identify chemical, radiological, and nuclear incidents. Physicians are generally too far away from the scene. In fact, physicians in clinics and hospitals rely heavily on reports provided by those at the incident site as they try to treat casualties.

Table 6 - Characteristics of agents

	Description	**Time of Effect Onset**	**Location of Diagnosis**
Chemical	Military or industrial chemical	Minutes	Field
Biological	Category A pathogens (anthrax, botulinum toxin, bubonic plague, hemorrhagic fever, smallpox, tularemia)	Hours to days	Medical facility
Radiological (Exposure device)	Exposes victims to clandestine radiation source.	Days to weeks or years	Medical facility
Radiological (Dispersal device)	Dirty bomb combines conventional explosives with radioactive material, typically low dose	Immediate explosion and opportunity to detect radiation	Field or medical facility
Nuclear	High dose radiation plus explosive dangers	Immediate or days	Field

CRESS is an acronym for symptoms related to chemical agents, including Consciousness, Respirations, Eyes, Secretions, and Skin. Clinical symptoms can differ depending upon the patient's underlying fitness and medical conditions. For example, surface agents like mustard may have systemic effects if the agent is absorbed quickly through a large skin wound. Similarly, chemical agents penetrate thin skin with dense underlying vasculature, such as on the scalp, much faster than thick skin with fewer blood vessels. Chemicals generally penetrate mucous membranes faster than they penetrate intact skin.

Table 7 - Chemical Agent Clinical Symptoms **(CRESS symptom list with antidote)**

Agent	**Conscious ness**	**Respira tions**	**Eyes**	**Secretions**	**Skin**	**Antidote**
Nerve (GA, GB, GD, VX), Russian Novichok agents	Depressed consciousness or unconscious, seizures	Increased	Constricted (miosis)	Increased (lacrimation, rhinorrhea, salivation, bronchial secretions)	Diaphoretic (cold and sweaty)	Atropine, Oximes, Diazepam
Cyanide (hydrogen sulfide, phosphine gas)	Depressed consciousness or unconscious	Increased	Normal	Normal, nausea	Flushed or cyanotic when shock is advanced	Oxygen, Vit B12, Sodium/amyl nitrite, sodium thiosulphate
Chlorine or Phosgene	Normal unless asphyxia causes a loss of consciousness	Increased, airway irritation	Normal, eye pain	Increased (lacrimation, rhinorrhea, salivation). Delayed fluid in lungs	Normal	Oxygen, rest (since phosgene symptoms worsen with exercise)
Vesicants (mustard, Lewisite, HF)	Normal	Increased if vapor, airway burns	Normal, inflamed or ulcerated if direct contact	Increased (lacrimation, rhinorrhea, salivation). Delayed fluid in lungs at very high doses.	Normal initially, red and blisters at up to 12-24 hours.	None
Opioid incapacitating agent (carfentanil)	Depressed consciousness or unconscious	Decreased	Constricted (miosis)	Normal	Normal	Narcan
Anti-cholinergic incapacitating agent	Agitated	Normal or increased	Normal or dilated (mydriasis)	Decreased	Hot and dry	Mad as a hatter, blind as a bat, dry as a bone, red as a beet, hot as hell[30]
Riot control agent	Normal	Normal or increased	Normal	Lacrimation, rhinorrhea, salivation	Normal	

The images below help visualize what chemical agents do to the bodies of their victims.

[30] Mad as a hatter refers to mental status changes, blind as a bat occurs because of dilated pupils, dry as a bone occurs because sweating is blocked, red as a beet is due to heat from inability to cool via perspiration, and hot as hell comes from the same reason.

Figure 5 – Clinical Findings of Chemical Exposure by Category[31]

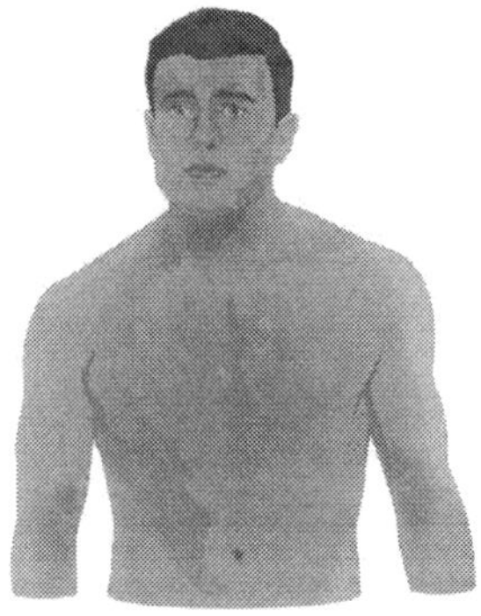	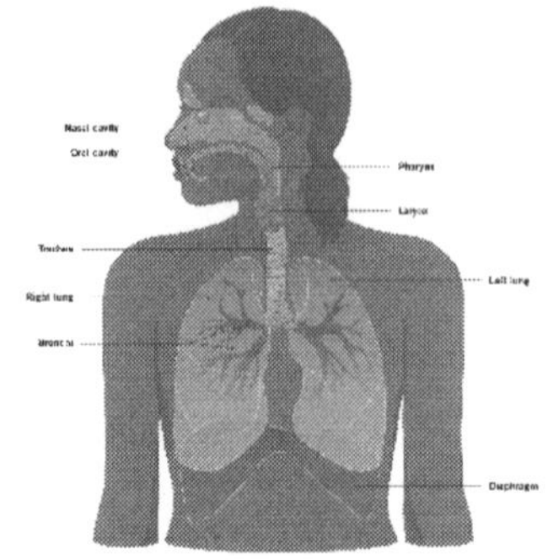	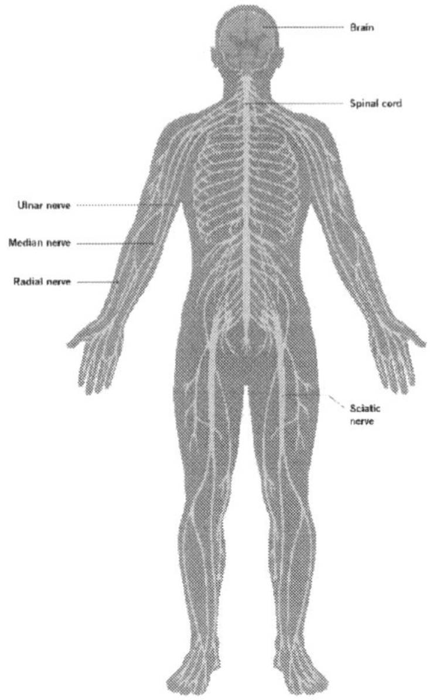
Blister Agents	Respiratory Agents	Nerve Agents

The most common field treatment for nerve agent exposure is Duodote, a mixture of atropine and 2 PAM chloride (Pralidoxime (2-pyridine aldoxime methyl chloride)). Duodote must be given as soon as possible after exposure, since agents "age" and effects become irreversible after minutes to hours, depending on the agent.

[31] Centers for Disease Control and Prevention, "Chemicals by Category," www.cdc.gov, April 4, 2022, https://www.cdc.gov/chemicalemergencies/hcp/chemicals-by-category.html.

Table 8 - Biological Agent Clinical Symptoms

	Symptoms	Notes
Anthrax[32]	1. Cutaneous and injection - painless skin ulcer, small bumps, and blisters 2. GI - dysphagia, nausea, vomiting, stomach pain, diarrhea, bloody GI fluids 3. Inhalational - fever, chills, chest pain, dyspnea, confusion, cough, headache,	Can progress from early symptoms to death in a matter of hours. Anthrax spores must be decontaminated but anthrax is not contagious person to person.
Botulinum Toxin[33]	Visual (blur, double, drooping eyelids, eyes hard to move), slurred speech, dyspnea, muscle weakness, dysphagia	Natural transmission in food or water. Aerosol distribution and inhalational botulism possible.
Bubonic Plague[34]	1. Bubonic – fever, headache, chills, weakness, swollen and painful lymph nodes. 2. Septicemic – bubonic symptoms, bleeding into skin, abdominal pain, shock 3. Pneumonic – dyspnea, chest pain, cough,	Death is likely in untreated cases, and pneumonic plague is transmissible person to person.
Hemorrhagic fever	Fever, headache, body aches, widespread unexplained bleeding, GI symptoms, sometimes jaundice and neurological symptoms.	Wide variety of viruses with varying symptoms.
Smallpox[35]	Fever, head and body aches, small red spots in mouth, pustular rash which scabs,	Eradicated but could return via intentional attack
Tularemia[36]	Painful ulcer at site where bacteria entered body, swollen and painful local lymph glands, high fever	Naturally occurring in animals

Responders to biological agent releases can also look for evidence of equipment and supplies to make or isolate the agent, such as machinery to produce anthrax spores. Transport containers and PPE are also important to note. The anthrax attack via the US mail in 2001 was done with a professional lab, but the perpetrator remains unknown.

The agents listed above are considered the most dangerous (Category A bioterrorism agents) by the US CDC. However, they are not the only agents which can be, or have been, used as

---

[32] "Anthrax," Centers for Disease Control and Prevention, 2020, https://www.cdc.gov/anthrax/. https://www.cdc.gov/anthrax/.

[33] "Botulism," Centers for Disease Control and Prevention, 2019, https://www.cdc.gov/botulism/.

[34] "Plague," Centers for Disease Control and Prevention, 2019, https://www.cdc.gov/plague/.

[35] "Smallpox," Centers for Disease Control and Prevention, 2019, https://www.cdc.gov/smallpox/.

[36] "Tularemia," Centers for Disease Control and Prevention, 2018, https://www.cdc.gov/tularemia/.

bioterror weapons. The largest bioterrorism attack in US history occurred when members of the Rajneesh Cult located outside the Dalles, a city in Oregon, spread salmonella in several salad bars in 1984. No one died, but 751 people became ill and 45 were hospitalized.[37] The motive for the attack was political: the cult wanted to have its candidates elected to county leadership, and tried to sicken voters who might vote against them.

Radiological Agent Clinical Symptoms

Radiation has many industrial and medical uses in the United States, so radiation sources are widespread, from factories to hospitals. Of the hundreds of types of sources, only a few would be practical to use in a "dirty bomb," a conventional explosive tainted with radioactive materials. These include americium-241, californium-252, caesium-137, cobalt-60, iridium-192, plutonium-238, polonium-210, radium-226 and strontium-90.

The primary injury would occur due to the bomb explosives, but the radiation could cause panic in the geographic area affected. Most patients would have a small enough dose of radiation to be asymptomatic, but a few could develop nausea, vomiting, fatigue, and loss of appetite. Acute radiation sickness (ARS) is unlikely in a dirty bomb situation.

---

[37] Gregory R Ciottone, *Disaster Medicine* (Philadelphia: Elsevier/Mosby, 2016), 732. Salmonella is a category B biothreat agent.

Figure 6 – Contamination and Exposure[38]

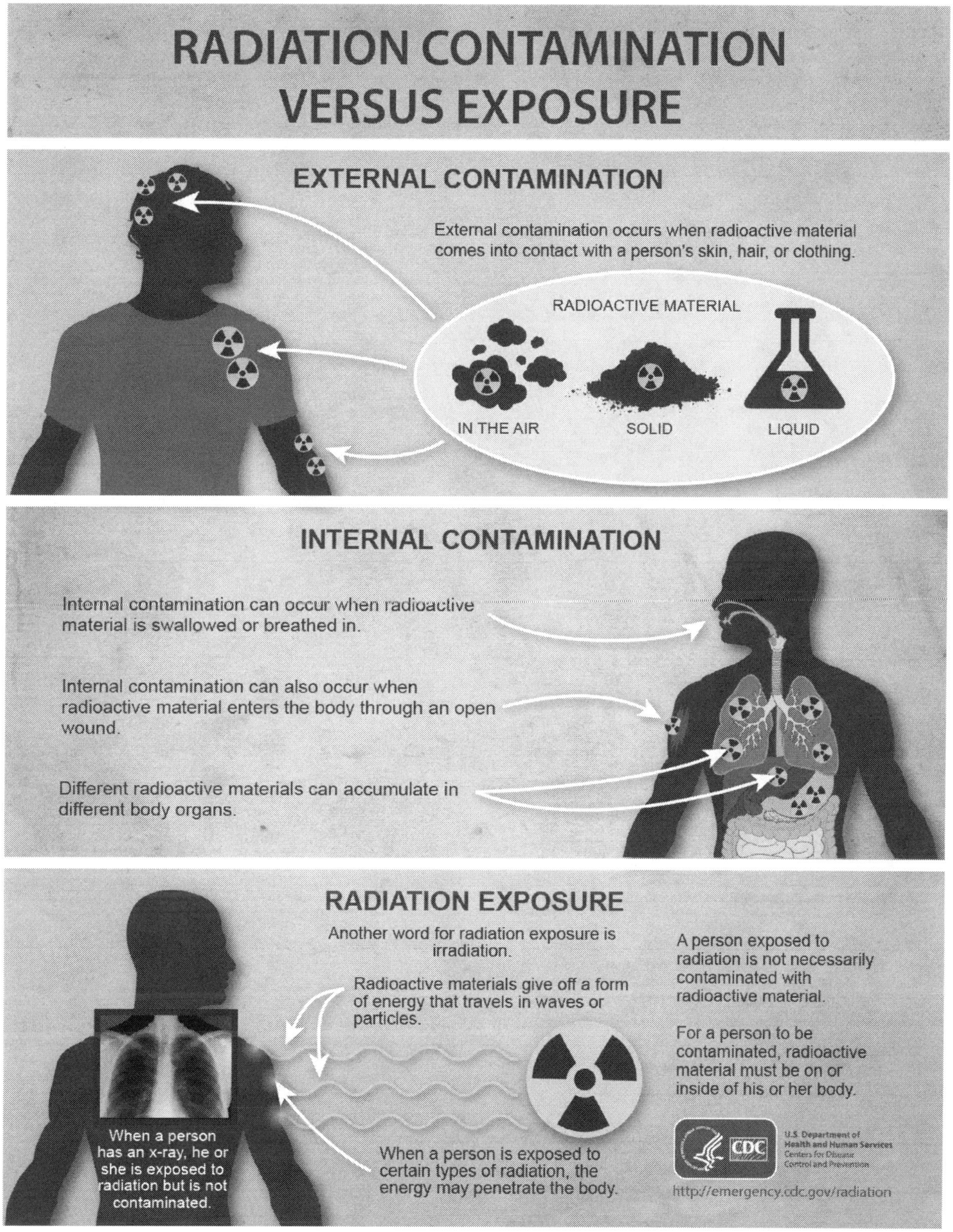

[38] "Radiation Contamination versus Exposure," Centers for Disease Control and Prevention, March 25, 2022, https://www.cdc.gov/nceh/radiation/emergencies/pdf/infographic_contamination_versus_exposure.pdf.

Figure 7 – Radiological exposure[39]

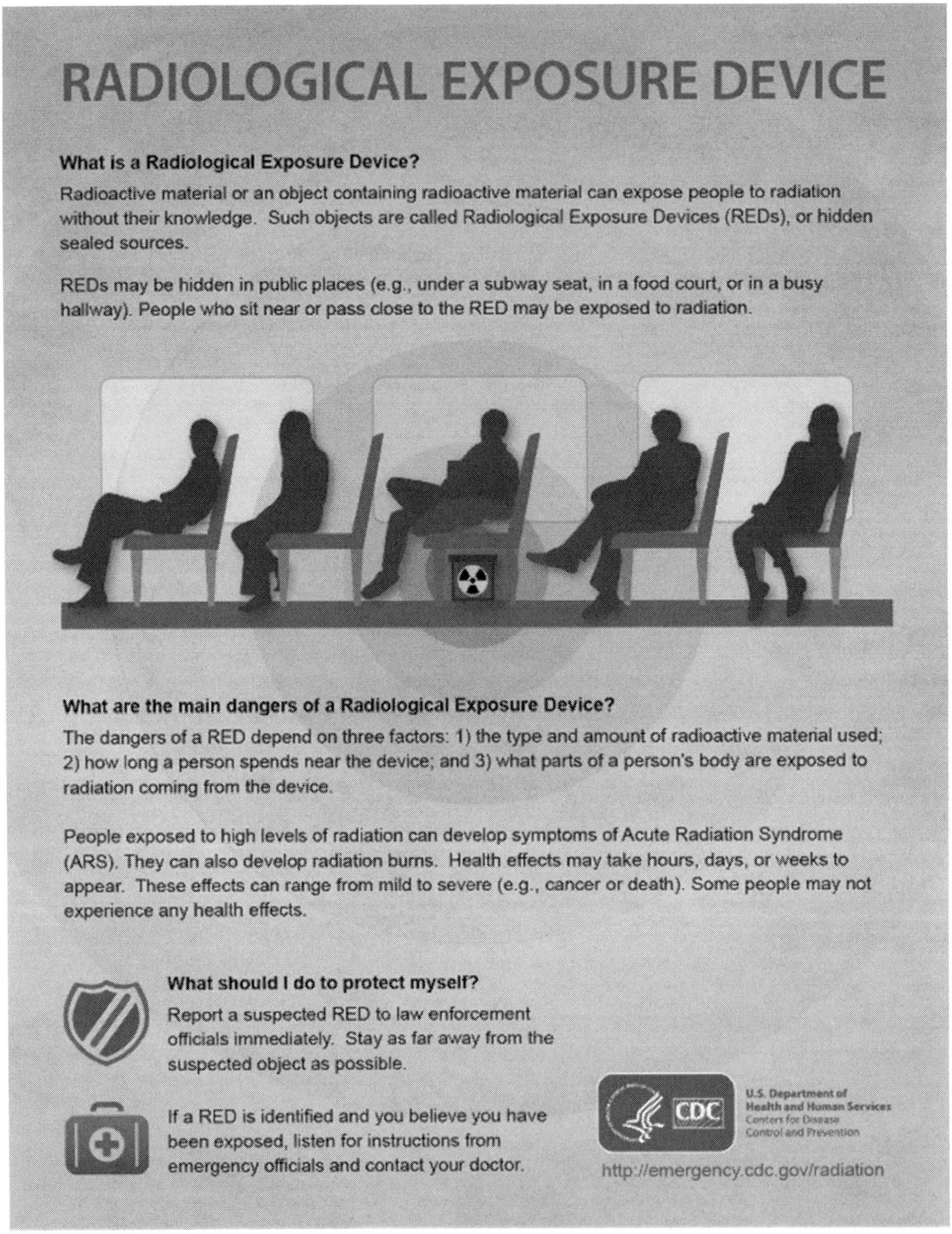

[39] "Radiological Exposure Device," Centers for Disease Control and Prevention, January 23, 2023, https://www.cdc.gov/nceh/multimedia/infographics/radiological_exposure_device.html.

Radiological sources are ubiquitous. In August 1994, a Boy Scout named David Hahn collected americium from smoke detectors, radium from clocks, tritium from gunsights, and thorium from the mantles of camping lanterns in the hopes of making a breeder reactor in a shed in his back yard. He failed to make a reactor, but did expose himself and others to high levels of radiation. Radiation sources are still found in a wide variety of consumer products.[40] Anyone with a modicum of knowledge and money could harvest enough radiation, along with explosives (such as black powder) or simple incendiaries (such as gasoline and sawdust), to make a low-grade radiological dispersal device.

[40] US EPA, "What Kinds of Consumer Products Contain Radioactive Materials?," US EPA, February 11, 2019, https://www.epa.gov/radiation/what-kinds-consumer-products-contain-radioactive-materials.

The Chernobyl Nuclear Reactor disaster in 1986 provides a useful case study. Due to mistakes during a routine test, reactor 4 exploded and the radioactive core melted down, releasing a large amount of radiation, including radioactive particles. The radiation particle cloud traversed Europe and the Middle East. One hundred thirty-four people developed acute radiation sickness (ARS) and 28 of those died of ARS. Over the next two decades, life expectancy declined from age 65 to age 58 in the areas near Chernobyl, but the deaths were not related to radiation. Instead, people died from depression, alcoholism, and suicide related to fear of radiation.[41]

In 1995, Chechen insurgents buried a conventional bomb contaminated with cesium 137 in a park in Moscow.[42] Three years later, a device with radioactive materials was found attached to an explosive mine near railroad tracks in Chechnya. Neither dirty bomb exploded, as the first was reported to the media and the second was discovered before detonation.

What would likely occur with a radiological dispersal device? A dirty bomb exploded outside the Humphrey Building (Health and Human Services – HHS) in Washington DC, for example, would damage the building and its surroundings. Depending upon where the bomb detonated, it could spew radioactive material to the US Capitol and the Rayburn House Office Building. The presence of radiation would cause the entire area to be blocked off until it was cleaned up, which could take weeks. Costs for cleanup and lost productivity would be high, even if no one died and there were few injured. Litigation costs would be astronomical.

---

[41] Gregory R Ciottone, *Disaster Medicine* (Philadelphia: Elsevier/Mosby, 2016), 616

[42] Gregory R Ciottone, *Disaster Medicine* (Philadelphia: Elsevier/Mosby, 2016), 462.

Figure 8 – Dirty Bomb/RDD[43]

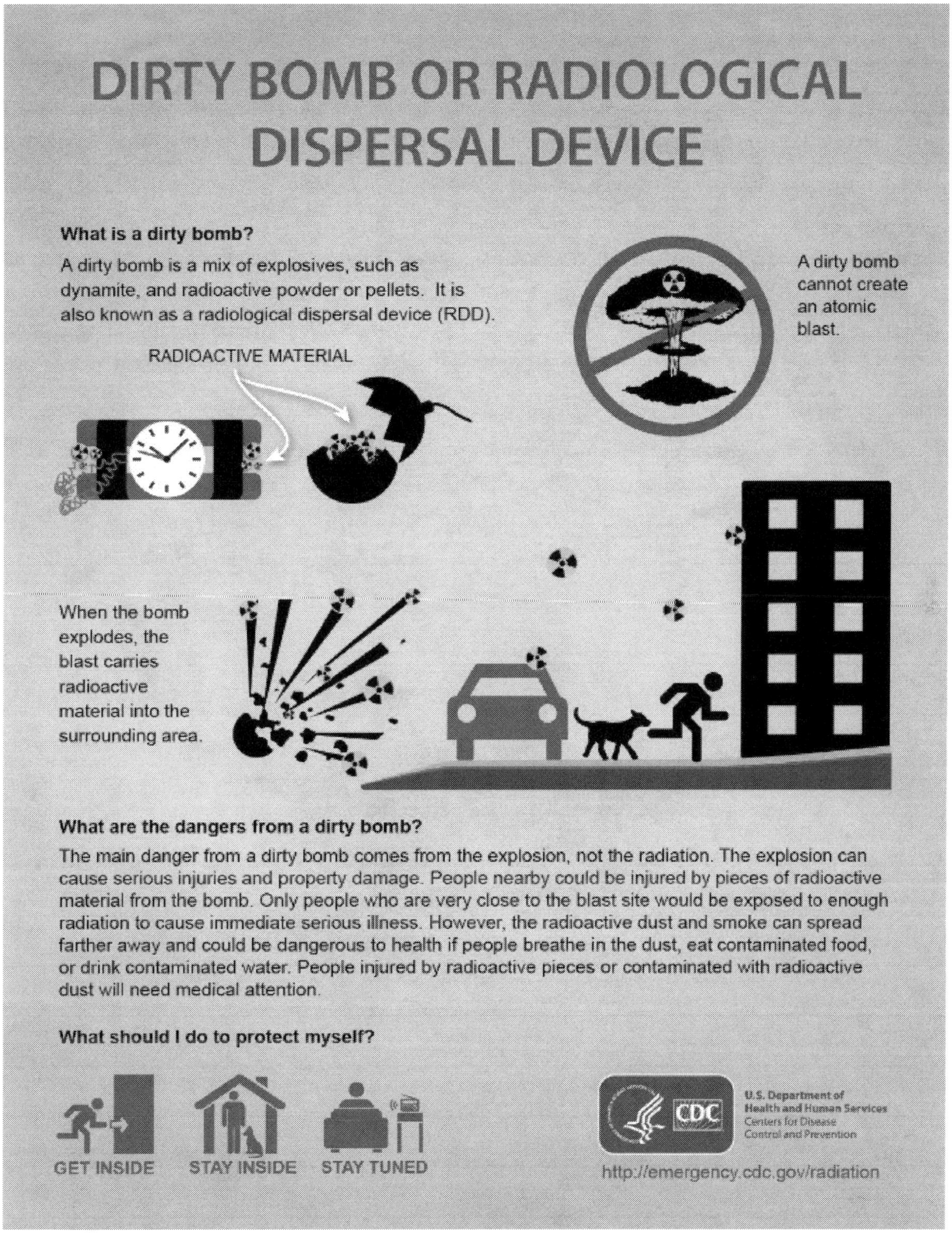

[43] "Dirty Bomb or Radiological Dispersal Device | Chemicals, Radiation and Toxicology Infographics | NCEH," Centers for Disease Control and Prevention, February 6, 2020, https://www.cdc.gov/nceh/multimedia/infographics/dirty_bomb_radiological_dispersal_device.html.

Nuclear Detonation Clinical Symptoms (blast and heat plus radiation)

At the height of the Cold War, the US and USSR had an estimated 40,000 nuclear warheads with the equivalent blasting power of 13,000 million tons of TNT.[44] Today, the US arsenal is smaller, as is the reported Russian arsenal, but China is building hundreds of nuclear weapons. Highly enriched radiation sources, the kind used for weapons, are smuggled throughout the world.

The anticipated scenario for a nuclear weapon, even a small one, detonated in any metropolis in the world is chilling. For example, a terrorist organization could detonate a 10 kt device hidden in a truck parked in downtown Manhattan.[45] Nearly everything and everyone within half a mile would be completely destroyed. Infrastructure at one and three miles would be significantly damaged. Immediate radioactive fallout would occur for the next twenty miles. Over 500,000 people would likely die.

Fission reactions, the foundation of atomic bombs, generate enormous amounts of energy. In a typical ground burst, such as a terrorist attack with the device in a parked truck, 50% of the energy is expended in the blast, 35% in thermal radiation (heat), 4% in initial ionizing radiation (first minute), 10% residual radiation (fallout), and 1% electromagnetic pulse (EMP).[46] In weapons of more than 10 kt, heat is the primary cause of injury.

Table 9 - Damage zones[47]

	Distance from ground zero	**Blast over-pressure**	**Effect**	**Medical**	**Response**
Severe	0.5 mile	5-8 psi	Buildings collapsed, streets impassible, few if any survivors.	Air emboli, Internal thoracic injuries, hemorrhage	Avoid this area unless rescuing confirmed survivors
Mod-erate	1 mile	2-5 psi	Only reinforced concrete buildings remain, utilities disrupted, fires	Ear drum rupture, people thrown against objects	Wear PPE. Limit time due to radiation.
Light	3 miles	0.5-2 psi	Windows and doors blown in, light construction destroyed		Primary injuries from flying glass and fragments.

[44] Gregory R Ciottone, *Disaster Medicine* (Philadelphia: Elsevier/Mosby, 2016), 462.

[45] The blast yield for atomic weapons is calculated as the equivalent amount of trinitrotoluene (TNT). A 10 kt atomic bomb has the same explosive power as 10,000 tons of TNT. For comparison, the "Little Boy" atomic device that destroyed Hiroshima was 15 kt, and the "Fat Man" bomb that obliterated Nagasaki was 21 kt.

[46] Gregory R Ciottone, *Disaster Medicine* (Philadelphia: Elsevier/Mosby, 2016), 621.

[47] Gregory R Ciottone, *Disaster Medicine* (Philadelphia: Elsevier/Mosby, 2016), 622

Rescuers and medical treatment personnel should be aware that thermal injury and radiation injuries look similar on exam. The primary difference is time. For example, heat burns from nuclear detonation occur instantly while burns from radiation do not appear for a few days.

Acute radiation sickness (ARS) has four phases.

1. Prodrome – nausea, vomiting, fatigue.
2. Latency – in general, patients whose vomiting begins before four hours after exposure have received a high dose of radiation.
3. Manifest illness – gastrointestinal, hematologic, cardiovascular, and central nervous system symptoms.
4. Outcome - Recovery or death. The lethal radiation dose for 50% of exposed people is 3.5 Gray (Gy).[48]

Beyond ARS, victims of radiation injuries should have long term surveillance for the development of malignancies and other complications. Psychological injury is common in nuclear survivors.

[48] A Gray is one of the two units used to measure the amount of radiation absorbed by an object or person, known as the "absorbed dose," which reflects the amount of energy that radioactive sources (with any type of ionizing radiation) deposit in materials (e.g., water, tissue, air) through which they pass. One gray (Gy) is the international system of units (SI) equivalent of 100 rads, which is equal to an absorbed dose of 1 Joule/kilogram. An absorbed dose of 0.01 Gy means that 1 gram of material absorbed 100 ergs of energy (a small but measurable amount) as a result of exposure to radiation. US Nuclear Regulatory Commission, https://www.nrc.gov/reading-rm/basic-ref/glossary/gray-gy.html.

Figure 9 – Shelter in a radiation emergency[49]

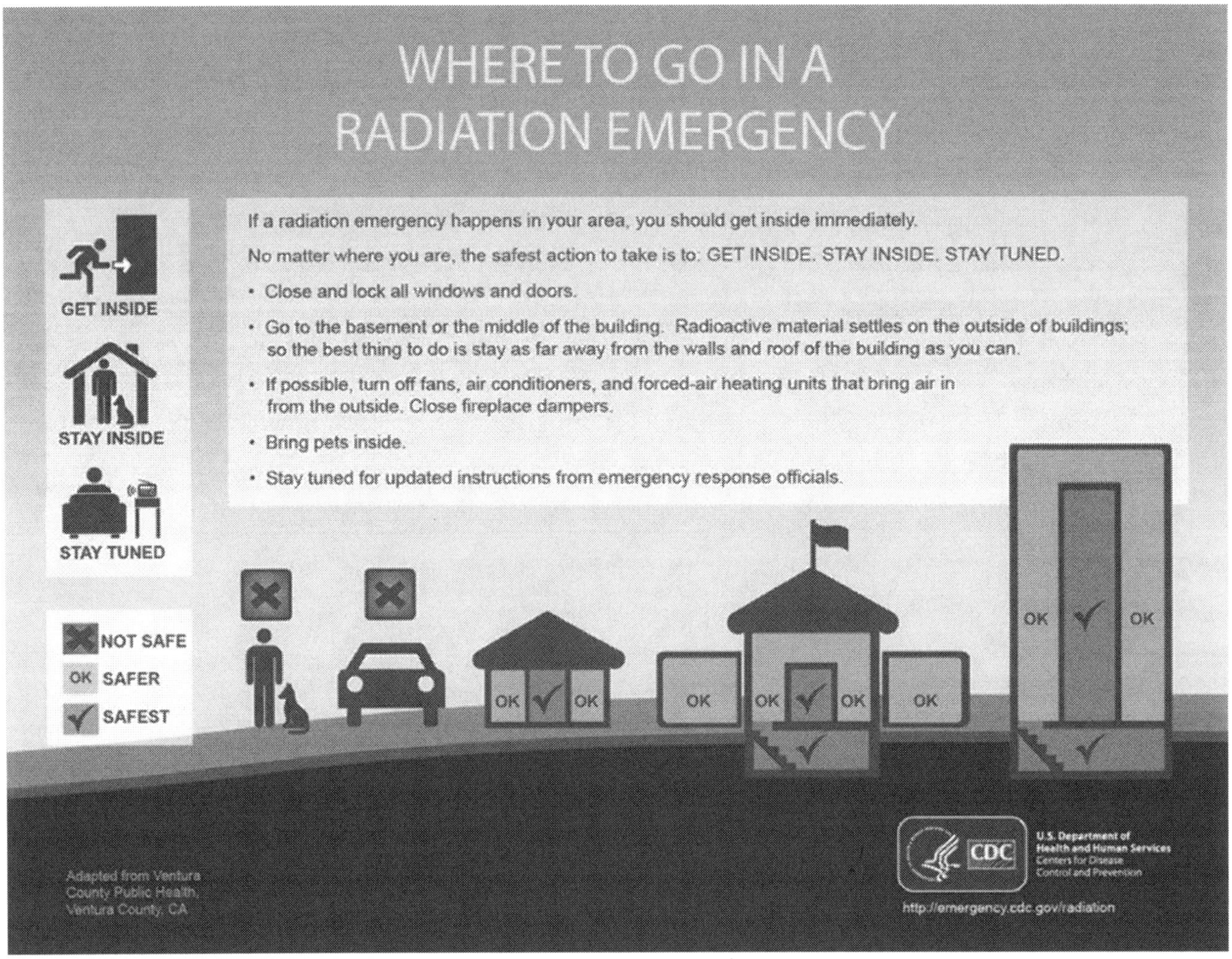

[49] "Where to Go in a Radiation Emergency | Chemicals, Radiation and Toxicology Infographics | NCEH," Centers for Disease Control and Prevention, February 6, 2020, https://www.cdc.gov/nceh/multimedia/infographics/radiation_emergency.html.

Figure 10 – Nuclear Weapon Hazards[50]

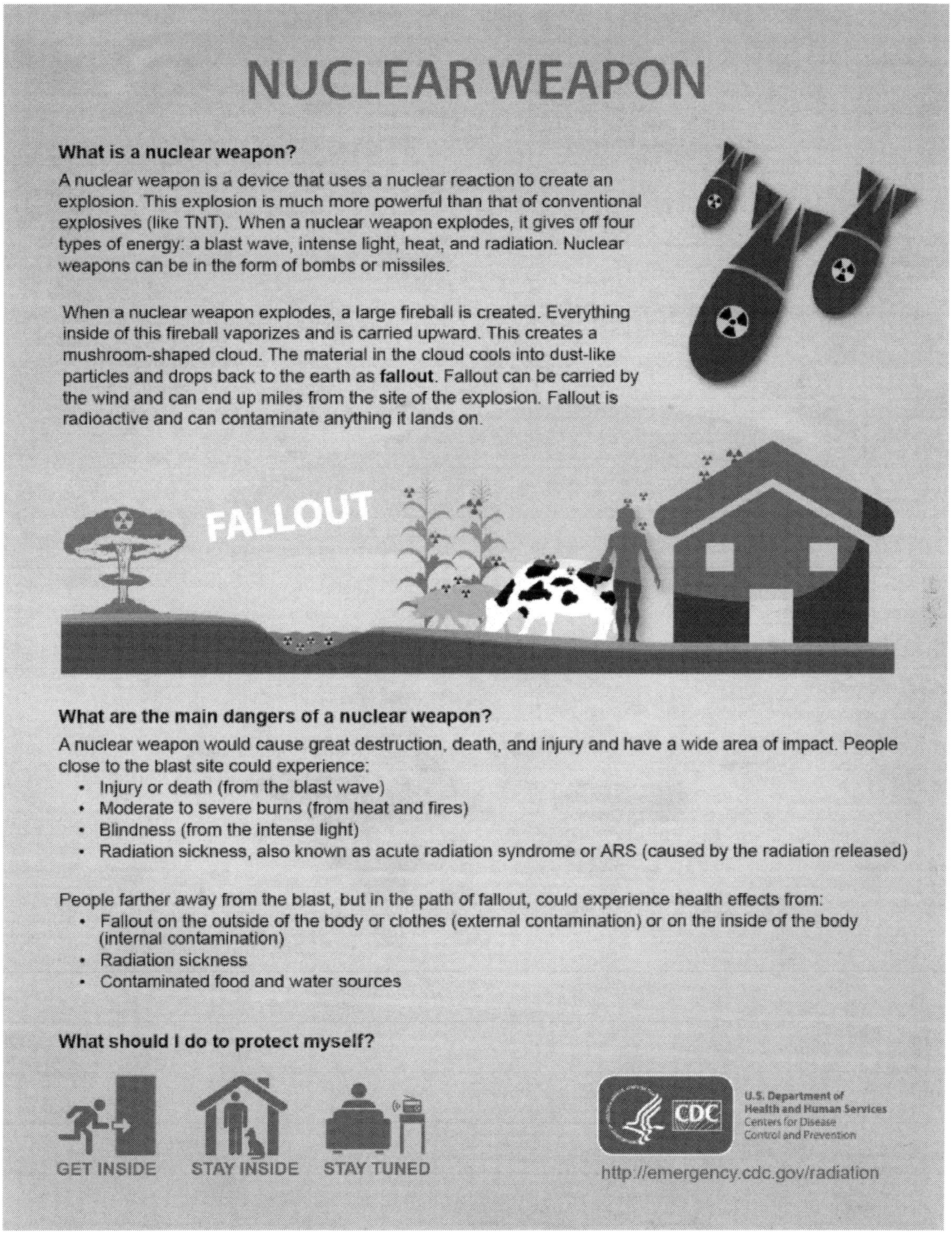

---

[50] Centers for Disease Control and Prevention, "Nuclear Weapon | Chemicals, Radiation and Toxicology Infographics | NCEH," Centers for Disease Control and Prevention, February 6, 2020, https://www.cdc.gov/nceh/multimedia/infographics/nuclear_weapon.html.

The effects of a nuclear weapon include the initial blast with heat in the millions of degrees, a blast wave, secondary shrapnel, and radiation. Total dose received from whole body radiation and the expected clinical and laboratory outcomes is described below.

Figure 11 – Triage with trauma and irradiation[51]

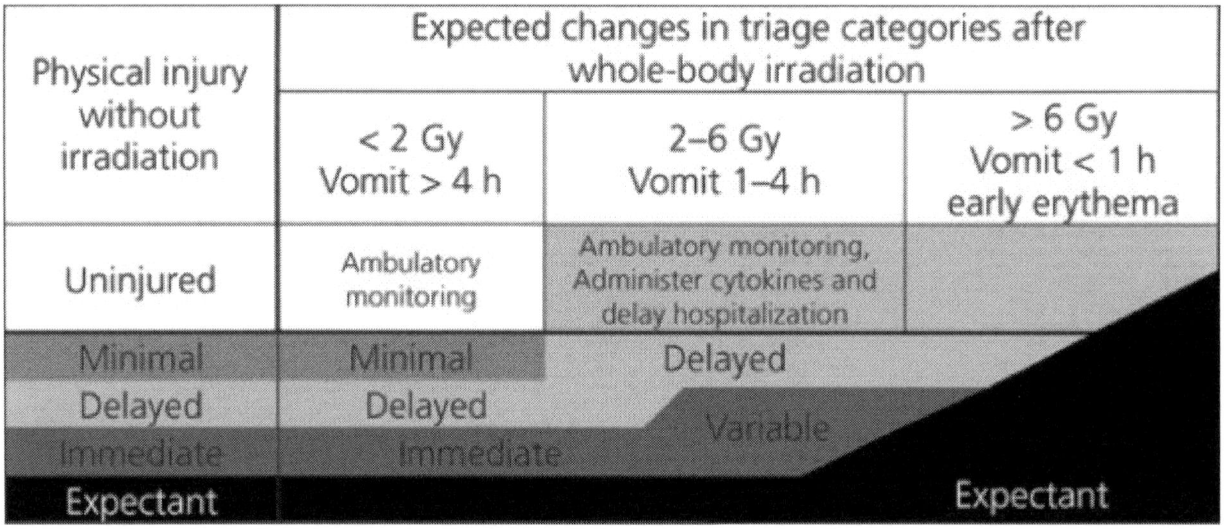

A patient is triaged by both his physical injury and his radiological exposure. Someone with an untreatable injury, given resources available, is expected to die regardless of radiation injury. Simultaneously, someone uninjured by the nuclear blast, heat, or shrapnel, who nonetheless received 12 Gy of radiation exposure, will almost certainly die.

[51] Armed Forces Radiobiology Research Institute, "MEDICAL MANAGEMENT of RADIOLOGICAL CASUALTIES" (Bethesda, MD: Military Medical Operations, July 2013), https://afrri.usuhs.edu/sites/default/files/2020-07/4edmmrchandbook.pdf.

Figure 12 – Symptoms and dosages after irradiation[52]

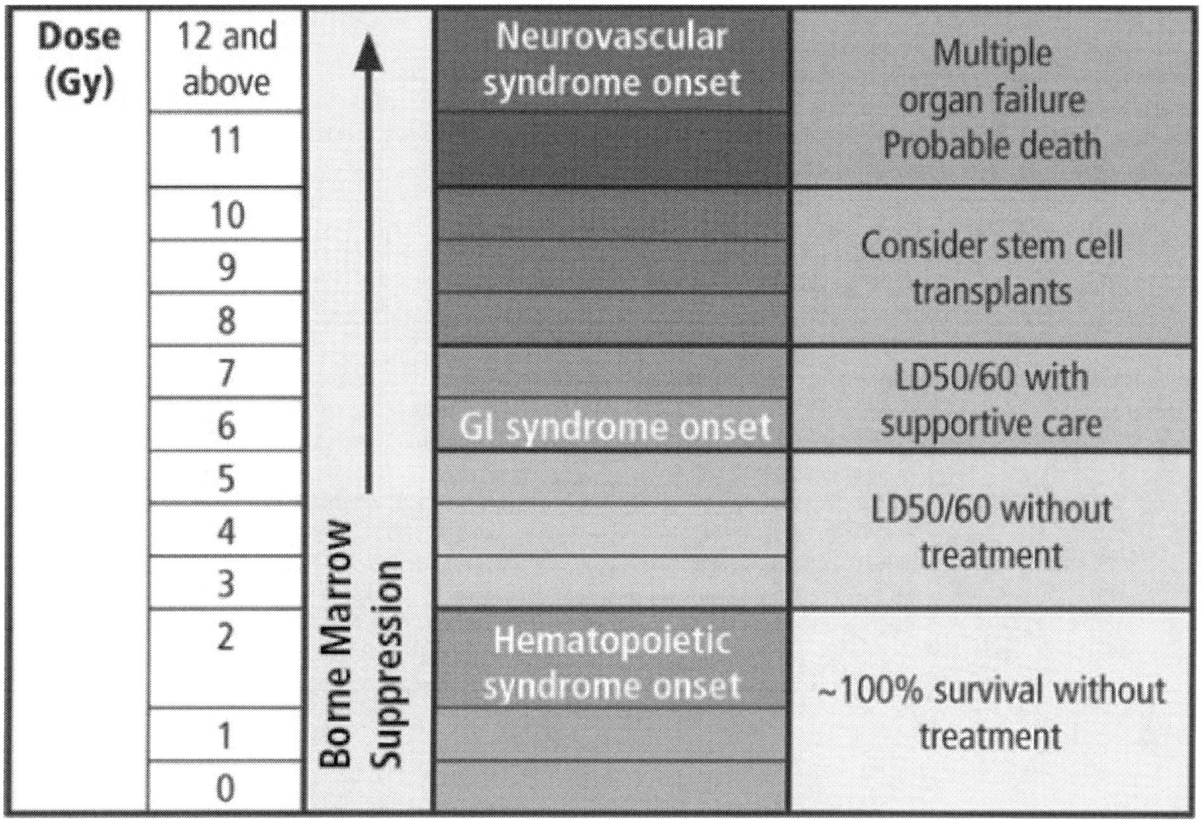

[52] Armed Forces Radiobiology Research Institute, "MEDICAL MANAGEMENT of RADIOLOGICAL CASUALTIES" (Bethesda, MD: Military Medical Operations, July 2013), https://afrri.usuhs.edu/sites/default/files/2020-07/4edmmrchandbook.pdf.

Figure 13 – Trends in Blood Tests after Irradiation[53]

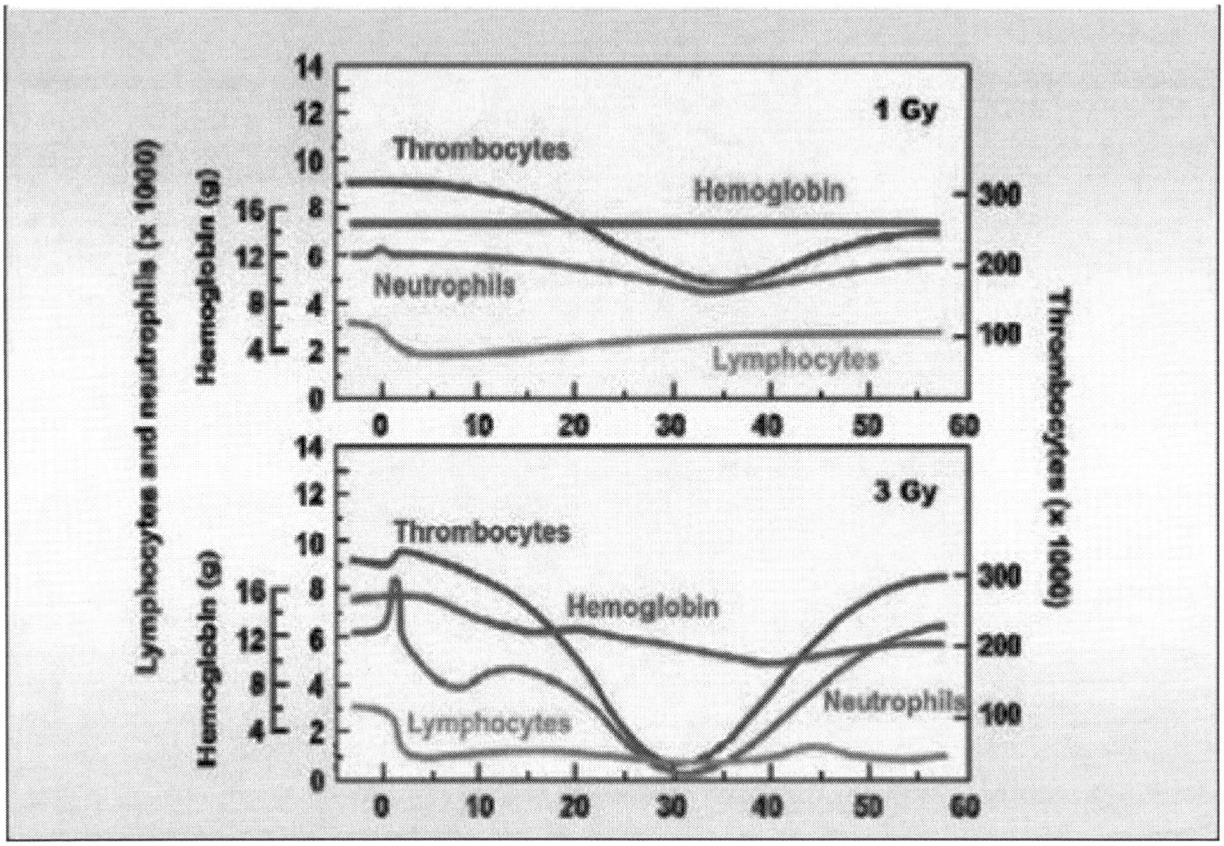

Treatment of Radiological Casualties

1. Treat conventional injuries first.
2. Supportive care – control of nausea, hydration, rest.
3. Prussian Blue - Reducing absorption by the human body in the case of internal injury.
4. Fluids – high fluid intake will dilute and aid in the biological elimination of some ingested radioactive agents.
5. Potassium iodide – block radiation from vulnerable tissues like the thyroid gland.
6. Oral phosphate – displace radioactive materials by non-radioactive materials.
7. Ammonium chloride – mobilize radioactive agent for faster elimination.
8. Ca/Zn DTPA – chelate radioactive material.
9. Specialty consultation – hematology, oncology, infectious disease, and radiation-trained personnel.

[53] Armed Forces Radiobiology Research Institute, "MEDICAL MANAGEMENT of RADIOLOGICAL CASUALTIES" (Bethesda, MD: Military Medical Operations, July 2013), https://afrri.usuhs.edu/sites/default/files/2020-07/4edmmrchandbook.pdf.

Chapter 6

CBRN Medical Incident Management

If a major chemical agent release or nuclear explosion happened in an uninhabited area of the Sahara Desert, the response would be muted. If the same thing happened in New Delhi, the response would be enormous. In the first case, few would be affected. In the latter, tens of thousands could die. This truth reminds us of our primary reason to be emergency responders, which is to save lives. Medicine, therefore, is a primary function of incident management. Management principles for a CBRN incident can be summarized as **SC_3AT_3ER** as explained below.

Safety – Responders must be in appropriate PPE. Non-responders must be excluded from the scene.

Cordons[54]

1. Hot – Area of direct exposure to hazard in the environment (WMD/CRNE, HAZMAT, firearm, explosive). If PPE does not mitigate the threat, it may be an exclusion zone.
    a. Self- and first aid
    b. Triage
    c. Casualty assessment ('quick look' include a trauma primary survey)
    d. Life-saving interventions (T1 casualties) for CBRN and trauma
    e. Evacuation to the Casualty Collection Point (CCP)
2. Warm – Area of decontamination between hot and cold zones. Clean/dirty line is between hot and warm zones.
    a. Triage
    b. Casualty assessment ('quick look' including Trauma Primary Survey)
    c. Life-saving interventions (T1 casualties)
    d. Casualty hazard management, e.g., decontamination
    e. Wound management
    f. Evacuation to the Casualty Clearing Station (CCS) or a medical treatment facility (MTF).
    g. For specific agents and depending on evacuation timelines, MedCM may be given to prevent the deterioration of T2/3 casualties.
3. Cold – Clean area inside outer cordon.
    a. Supportive care
    b. Definitive care

---

[54] Steven A. Bland, "Chemical, Biological, Radiological and Nuclear (CBRN) Casualty Management Principles," *Conflict and Catastrophe Medicine*, November 22, 2013, 747–70, https://doi.org/10.1007/978-1-4471-2927-1_46.

Command and Communication – each zone has its own chain of command which is integrated into the overall chain of command for the incident. Leaders from general services (fire, police, EMS), and specialist services (HAZMAT) coordinate and communicate at lower and higher levels. The overall incident command may be as much as 3,000 feet from the hazard location.[55]

Assessment – Ongoing environmental and casualty assessments.

Triage

1. Immediate (need help immediately but can survive if help is provided and adequate resources are available)
2. Delayed (can survive delay of up to four hours)
3. Minimal (walking wounded)
4. Expectant (unsavable due to severity of condition given available resources)

Treatment – Definitive treatment occurs after decontamination if such is necessary.

Transport - Definitive transport occurs after decontamination if such is necessary.

Exploitation and Recovery – Return resources consumed to functional status or replace them.

---

[55] International Association of Fire Chiefs and National Fire Protection Association, *Fundamentals of Fire Fighter Skills and Hazardous Materials Response* (Burlington, MA: Jones & Bartlett Learning, 2020), 1149.

Figure 14- Prussian Blue[56]

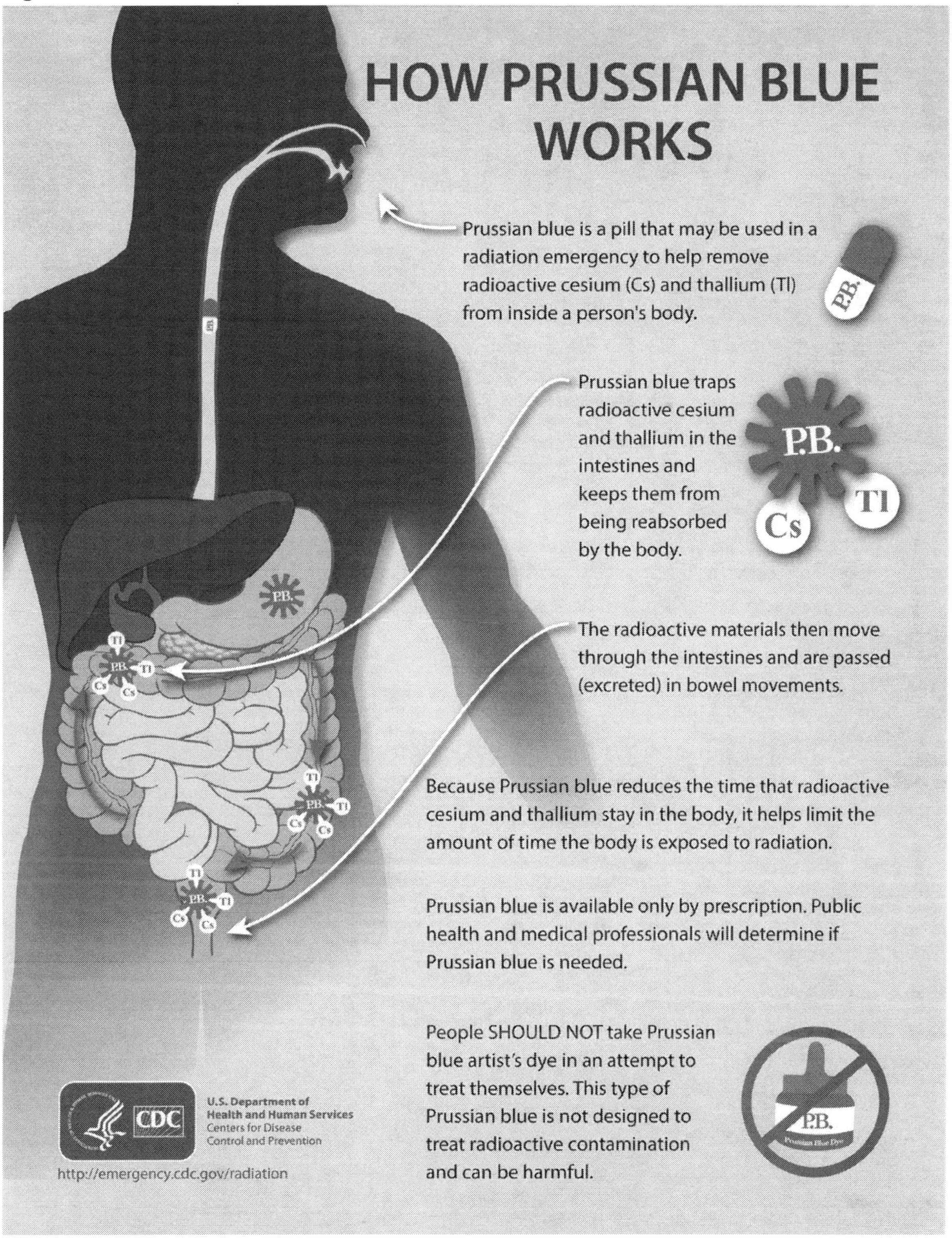

[56] "CDC Radiation Emergencies | Facts about Prussian Blue," Centers for Disease Control and Prevention, April 25, 2019, https://www.cdc.gov/nceh/radiation/emergencies/prussianblue.htm.

Figure 15 – Potassium Iodide[57]

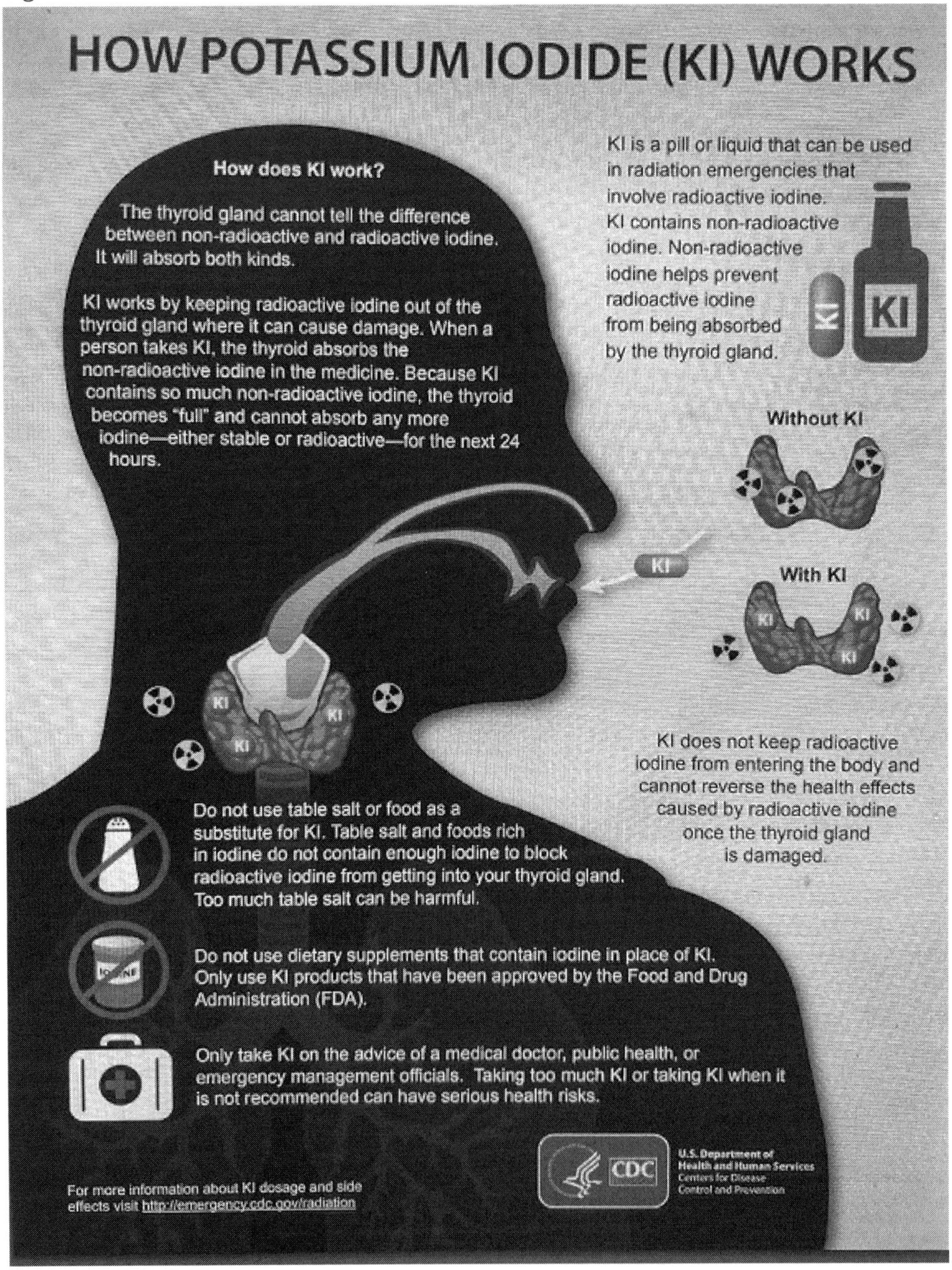

[57] "How Potassium Iodide (KI) Works," *Centers for Disease Control and Prevention*, n.d., https://www.cdc.gov/nceh/radiation/emergencies/pdf/infographic_ki.pdf.

Casualty Management

The ABCDE mnemonic used in BLS, ACLS, ATLS, and other protocols is useful for immediate treatment of life-threatening injuries and exposures.

1. If the incident is confirmed as CBRN, use PPE and consider how to contain the problem.
2. Establish containment zones (hot, warm, and cold).
3. **A**irway management and antidotes
4. **B**reathing - cyanosis, respiratory distress, tension pneumothorax, or sucking chest wound.
5. **C**irculation – severe hemorrhage, shock, bradycardia from nerve agent.
6. **D**isability (neurological) and decontamination – unconsciousness or convulsions.
7. **E**xposure (manage patient temperature, expose or cover as appropriate) and evacuation to more permissive environment.

Interventions for Life Threatening Conditions

1. Triage and provide lifesaving treatment to affected personnel in the hot zone. Evacuate.
2. Apply tourniquet(s)
3. Apply a pressure dressing and hemostatic agents.
4. Basic airway management including suction **(A)**
5. Administer early MedCM/antidote administration including anticonvulsant.
6. Ventilate (as resources allow) **(B)**
7. Administer oxygen **(B)**
8. Manage tension pneumothorax, such as needle decompression **(B).**
9. Manage sucking chest wound, such as application of dressing with valve **(B)**
10. Resuscitation with fluids (trauma, sepsis, or combined injuries) **(C)**
11. Manage severe sepsis and septic shock (fluids, oxygen, and antibiotics) **(C)**
12. Remove from the hazard (self-extraction or rescue)
13. If the hazard is radiological or chemical, decontaminate. If it is biological, isolate, including quarantine for the well and isolation for the ill.

Medical isolation is a standard procedure for hospitals and other health care facilities. Therefore, it will not be discussed here.

The overall goal for all victims is to stabilize any serious injuries, decontaminate them to minimize the doses of agent to which they are exposed, and decontaminate to protect others. This includes personnel (including rescuers, hospital personnel, etc.) and equipment (like the ambulance they will ride in). Transport patients quickly and safely to definitive care.

Chapter 7

Decontamination[58]

Separating "the person from the danger" is the watch phrase for most, if not all, emergency response. Occupational health professionals advise company leaders to engineer tasks so as to eliminate danger to workers. Firefighters drag or carry victims out of burning buildings. Police separate feuding parties to try to prevent them from hurting each other.

Likewise, decontamination separates the toxic agent - chemical, biological, or radiological - from the person the agent is endangering. There are two types, physical and chemical.

Physical removal – the mechanical removal of contaminants is one of the most effective means of protecting victims (from getting larger and larger doses), responders (from being exposed), and others. Physical removal includes the following:

1. Clothing removal
2. Irrigation with water – Dilutes and washes away the agent. Runoff water is contaminated and must be gathered and treated.
3. Detergents and soaps – Help water to dilute and wash away the agent. Both may slowly destroy chemical agents through hydrolysis.
4. Use of dry adsorbents – these adsorb liquid contamination. Examples include baking powder and Fuller's Earth. The adsorbents do not destroy the agent, only contain it, so off-gassing remains an issue.

Chemical Destruction – Some agents can be deactivated by altering their structure rather than simply diluting them or adsorbing them.

1. High temperature steam can remove grease and oil, which can hold contaminants. It can also sterilize and disinfect, de-ice, and kill algae and mildew.
2. Hot air can eliminate CBRN agents from nonporous and nonabsorbent surfaces.
3. Weathering uses natural forces (UV light, wind, water) to slowly decontaminate vehicles and other equipment through evaporation, hydrolysis, and photolysis.
4. Surfactants (especially anionic) – solubilize contaminants into an aqueous solution.
5. Oxidizing agents (calcium hypochlorite (Ca(OCl)2), sodium hypochlorite (NaOCl).
6. Chloramine-B (C6H5ClNNaO2S) (Neomagnol) comes in a towelette and can detoxify VX.
7. Strong bases, such as CaO, Ca(OH)2, sodium hydroxide (NaOH), and potassium hydroxide (KOH) can detoxify GA, GB, and GD.
8. DS2 is a general-purpose reactive decontaminant.
9. Microemulsions such as C8 are effective in the decontamination of VX, G agents, and HD.

---

[58] "Introduction to CB Decontaminants," www.ojp.gov (OJP, n.d.), accessed August 2, 2023.

Many of the specific decontaminants listed here are useful for vehicles or other equipment but not for patients. Check before using any chemical on a patient.

Figure 16 – MARCHE Summary[59]

TCCC + CBRN = (MARCHE)^2			
	Hot Zone	Warm Zone	Cold Zone
Priorities	• Think Care Under Fire, sometimes agent is like effective fire • "What is killing the casualty now, is it the agent or trauma?" The answer to this question dictates your treatments • Triage • Treat only immediate life-threats • Expose only what is needed to save life. • CRESS assessment. Identify nerve agent exposure. • If chemical contamination of a wound is suspected, expose perform rapid spot decontamination as soon as possible • Protect yourself and the casualty from the threat: time, distance, shielding, upwind, uphill, upstream • Heat injury from operating in PPE is common and may be unrelated to the agent. • Getting to the warm zone may require prolonged movement of the casualty. • A medic caring for chemical casualties is contaminated (dirty medic) and cannot cross to cold zone with patient until decontaminated. • In conventional TCCC, only massive hemorrhage is addressed during CUF. However, some chemical agents are rapid killers. Nerve agent antidotes and rapid decontamination must be administered as early as possible.	• Think Tactical Field Care • "What is killing the casualty now, is it the agent or trauma?" The answer dictates your treatments • Triage • Provide only life-saving care, get them to the cold zone for definitive care. • Replace dirty tourniquets and decontaminate indwelling devices or replace as indicated. • Casualty may require advanced airway management and ventilator support • Perform cutout and thorough decontamination. • Perform treatments while decontamination is being conducted. "Expose to treat". • Assess circulation and administer resuscitation fluids per TCCC guidelines only if absent radial pulse • Countermeasures: administer specific treatments for life-threats as needed based on exposure and symptoms • Hypothermia is a threat due to exposure during decontamination. • Determine whether altered mental status is due to chemical agent or trauma	• Think Tactical Evacuation or Prolonged Field Care • "What is killing the casualty now, is it the agent or trauma?" The answer to this question dictates your treatments. • Triage • Anticipate and mitigate hypothermia. • Receiving medical personnel may have little to no experience with CBRN. Ensure effective patient handoff. • Clean Medic (remains on cold zone side of hot line and not exposed to contaminated casualties)
TCCC	M: Massive Hemorrhage	M.A.R.: reassessment	(MARCHE)^2 reassessment
	A: Airway, assess	C: Circulation and Shock Status	
	R: Respirations, assess	H: Hyperthermia, H: Head Wounds (altered mental status	
	E: Extraction	E: Evacuation	
CBRN	M: Don Mask, Mask check	M.A.R.: reassessment	(MARCHE)^2 reassessment
	A: Antidote (ATNAA/CANA)	C: Countermeasures (drips, nebulized medicines, etc.)	
	R: Rapid Shot Decontamination	H: Hyperthermia, H: Head Wounds (altered mental status	
	E: Extraction	E: Evacuation	

Decontamination must be approached from a leader's perspective, but also how to actually do it from an individual victim or rescuer's perspective.

[59] https://jts.health.mil/index.cfm/PI_CPGs/cpgs.

Figure 17 - Decontamination[60]

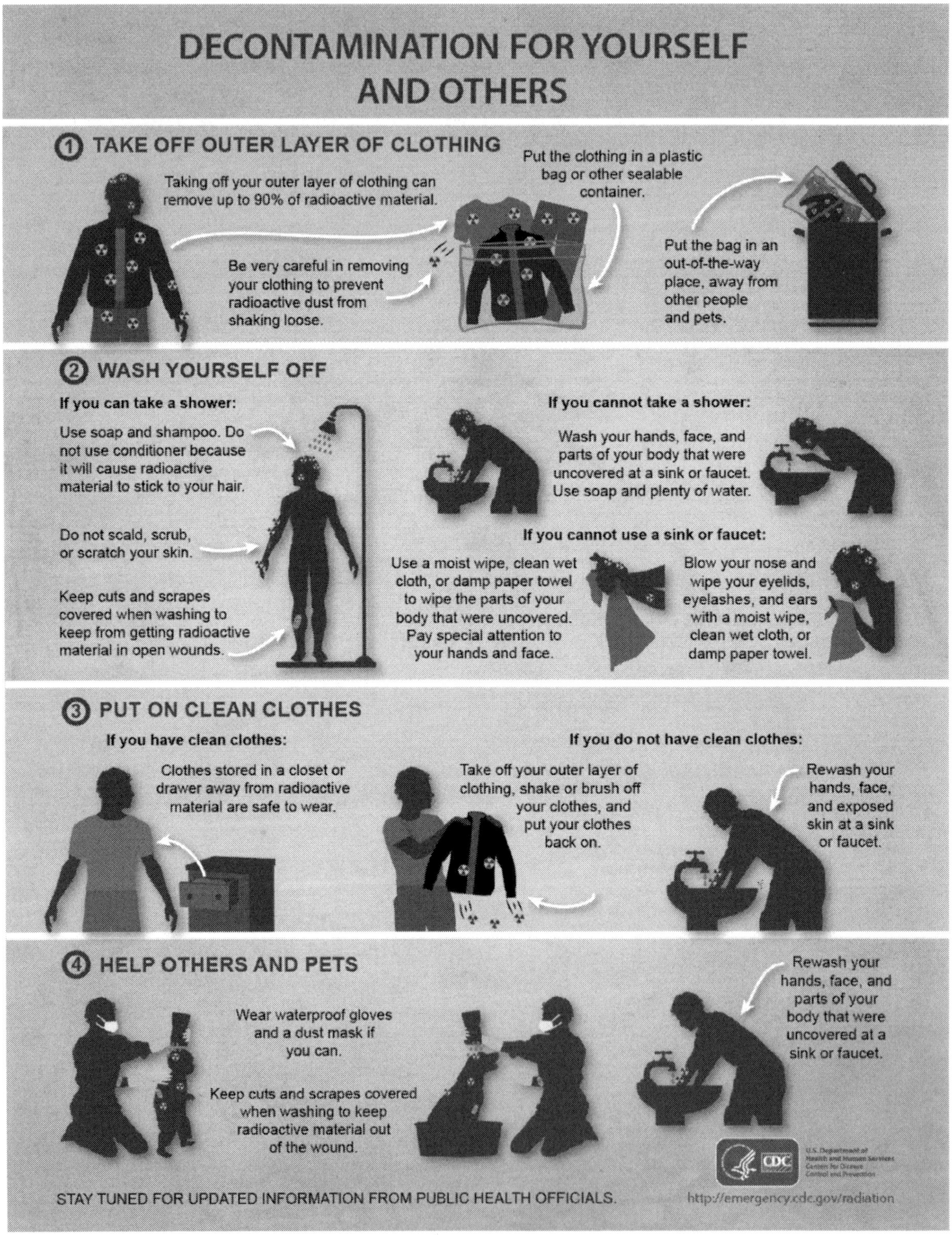

[60] "Decontamination for Yourself and Others," Centers for Disease Control and Prevention, February 6, 2020, https://www.cdc.gov/nceh/multimedia/infographics/decontamination.html.

Setting up a good decontamination site requires planning, equipment, supplies, personnel, and practice.

Figure 18 – Concept Diagram of an Emergency Response and Decontamination Site[61]

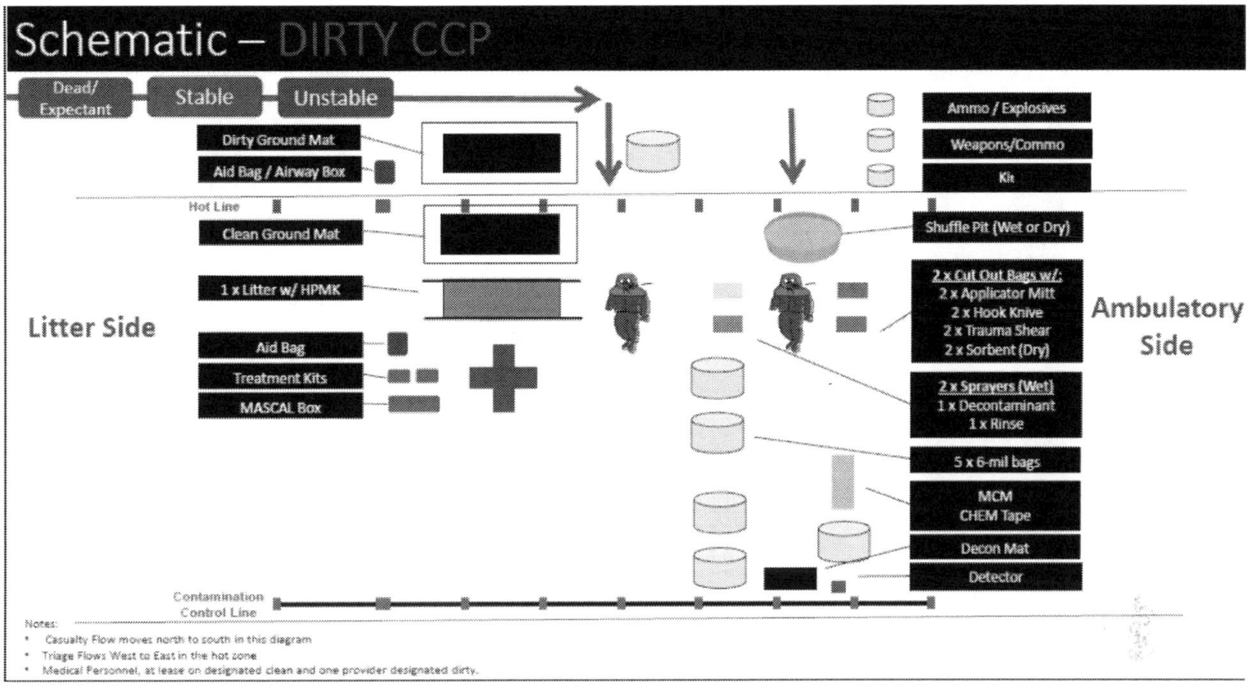

[61] George Barbee et al., "Joint Trauma System Clinical Practice Guideline: Chemical, Biological, Radiological and Nuclear (CBRN) Injury" (The Department of Defense Center of Excellence for Trauma, May 1, 2018), https://jts.health.mil/assets/docs/cpgs/Chemical_Biological,_Radiological_Nuclear_Injury_Part1_Initial_Response_01_May_2018_ID69.pdf.

Chapter 8

Critical Task List in WMD/CRBN/HAZMAT response and reset

It is not enough for first responders, facility-based medical personnel, leaders, and others to respond appropriately to a WMD/CBRN/HAZMAT event – they must respond effectively to the next one, and the next one. A system which handles a disaster or attack well but destroys itself in the process is no system at all. Further, the same people, equipment, supplies, and procedures which handle the rare WMD/CBRN/HAZMAT events must respond to the common structure fires, domestic disturbance calls, and heart attacks. In our limited resource world, we must build and maintain a system capable of handling the ordinary and of expanding and morphing to handle the extraordinary.

The following points will guide leaders as they consider not only how to make but also how to sustain an appropriate WMD/CBRN/HAZMAT response.

Protecting the responder(s)

1. Recognize WMD/CBRN/HAZMAT exposure requiring action to protect oneself and others.
2. Don personal protective equipment (PPE) and inform other responders to do the same.
3. Escape the threat, moving upwind, upstream, or uphill and utilize time, distance and shielding for protection when possible.

Protecting casualties

1. Recognize signs and symptoms of CBRN exposure that require immediate treatment of self and/or others. Chemical agent exposure is one example.
2. Prevent contamination of uncontaminated personnel, equipment, and facilities.
3. Consider all injuries, CBRN and otherwise, and address. For example, the DoD uses the Tactical Combat Casualty Care Card (TCCC) for clinical evaluation and documentation (TCCC + CBRN = MARCHE)
4. MARCHE = Massive hemorrhage/Mask, Airway/Antidote, Respiration/Rapid Spot Decontamination, Circulation/Countermeasure, Hypothermia/Head Injury, Extraction/Evacuation
5. Triage and treatment involve both TCCC and CBRN injuries in order of severity based on survivability and resources available.
6. Transportation
    a. Thorough decontamination prior to transport.
    b. Medical regulation to determine appropriate treatment facility.
    c. Warm hand-off of patient from emergency medical service to accepting provider.

Protecting the system

1. Reset equipment, supplies, and personnel to accept the next patient.
2. Identify and communicate lessons learned from prior events.
3. Begin comprehensive preincident planning for next event.
4. Train and equip.
5. The military acronym DOTMLPF is helpful – Doctrine, Organization, Training, Materiel (equipment and supplies), Leadership, Personnel, Facilities

Preincident Planning[62]

1. All organizations involved in WMD/CBRN/HAZMAT response must perform pre-incident planning.
2. Identify and quantify HAZMAT/WMD/CBRN hazards in the area (radiation sources, toxic chemicals). These can be naturally occurring (floods), technologically derived (airplane crash), or human-made (terror).
3. Identify resources that would be helpful in a disaster or terrorist event before the event.
4. Estimate the probability, location, and seasonality of various types of events.
5. Quantify human, property, and business impacts.

Training and Planning Considerations

1. Know how to do rapid spot and whole-body decontamination.
2. Required PPE – specialized and HAZMAT. Normal turnout SCBA is insufficient for a WMD/CBRN/HAZMAT environment. Use "CBRN certified SCBA" instead.
3. Field expedient PPE – Skin (nitrile gloves x 3), Equipment (6mm sheeting and bags).

Health and Safety Program to support WMD/CBRN/HAZMAT operations.

1. Medical surveillance, including pre-employment screening and periodic medical exams.
2. Response plans, including triage, treatment, and transportation, for acute, on-scene illness and injury.
3. HIPAA compliant record keeping.
4. Periodic review.

Legal Pitfalls and Risks in Emergency and Disaster Response[63]

1. Standards of practice and standards of medical care apply to emergency and disaster response situations just as they apply to more common situations. Gross negligence or willful malfeasance will cost a responder a bundle or put him or her in jail.
2. Organizations must develop and carry out a rapid response plan.

---

[62] Gregory R Ciottone, *Disaster Medicine* (Philadelphia: Elsevier/Mosby, 2016), 133-134.
[63] Gregory R Ciottone, *Disaster Medicine* (Philadelphia: Elsevier/Mosby, 2016), 81.

3. Responders, including volunteers and professionals, can be held personally liable for damages in a disaster situation.
4. No responders should act outside their scope of expertise during disaster response.
5. Responders must properly acknowledge and coordinate with chains of command and jurisdictional authorities. They must also act within the framework of federal and state disaster management plans.
6. Being aware of applicable laws and regulations, and training and preparing for a deployment to a disaster area, is essential.

Figure 19 – Sample triage and treatment card[64]

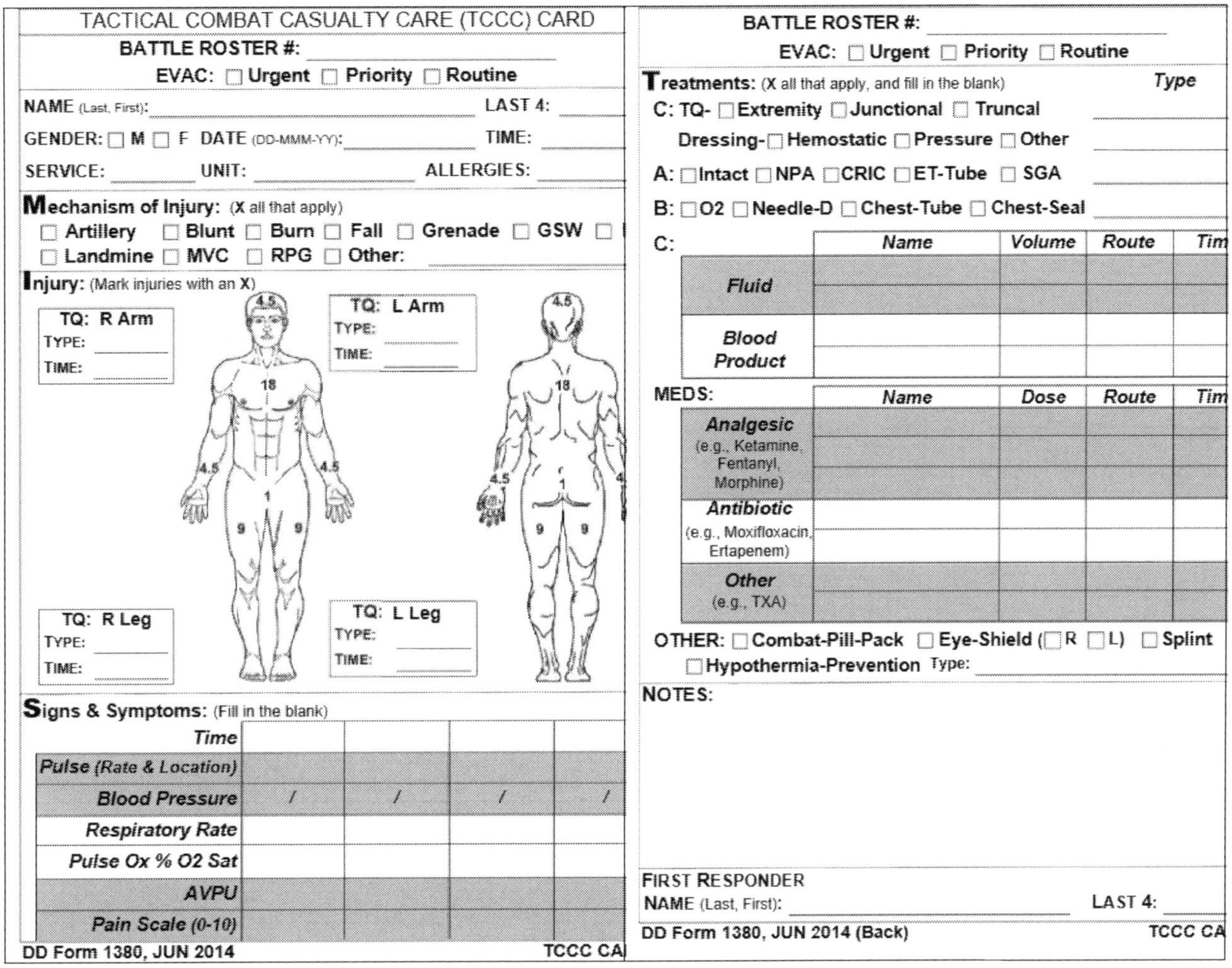

TACTICAL COMBAT CASUALTY CARE (TCCC) CARD

BATTLE ROSTER #: ____

EVAC: ☐ Urgent ☐ Priority ☐ Routine

NAME (Last, First): ____ LAST 4: ____

GENDER: ☐ M ☐ F DATE (DD-MMM-YY): ____ TIME: ____

SERVICE: ____ UNIT: ____ ALLERGIES: ____

Mechanism of Injury: (X all that apply)

☐ Artillery ☐ Blunt ☐ Burn ☐ Fall ☐ Grenade ☐ GSW ☐

☐ Landmine ☐ MVC ☐ RPG ☐ Other: ____

Injury: (Mark injuries with an X)

TQ: R Arm TYPE: ____ TIME: ____

TQ: L Arm TYPE: ____ TIME: ____

TQ: R Leg TYPE: ____ TIME: ____

TQ: L Leg TYPE: ____ TIME: ____

Signs & Symptoms: (Fill in the blank)

Time				
Pulse (Rate & Location)				
Blood Pressure	/	/	/	/
Respiratory Rate				
Pulse Ox % O2 Sat				
AVPU				
Pain Scale (0-10)				

DD Form 1380, JUN 2014 TCCC CA

BATTLE ROSTER #: ____

EVAC: ☐ Urgent ☐ Priority ☐ Routine

Treatments: (X all that apply, and fill in the blank) *Type*

C: TQ- ☐ Extremity ☐ Junctional ☐ Truncal ____

Dressing- ☐ Hemostatic ☐ Pressure ☐ Other ____

A: ☐ Intact ☐ NPA ☐ CRIC ☐ ET-Tube ☐ SGA ____

B: ☐ O2 ☐ Needle-D ☐ Chest-Tube ☐ Chest-Seal ____

C:

	Name	*Volume*	*Route*	*Tim*
Fluid				
Blood Product				

MEDS:

	Name	*Dose*	*Route*	*Tim*
Analgesic (e.g., Ketamine, Fentanyl, Morphine)				
Antibiotic (e.g., Moxifloxacin, Ertapenem)				
Other (e.g., TXA)				

OTHER: ☐ Combat-Pill-Pack ☐ Eye-Shield (☐ R ☐ L) ☐ Splint

☐ Hypothermia-Prevention Type: ____

NOTES:

FIRST RESPONDER

NAME (Last, First): ____ LAST 4: ____

DD Form 1380, JUN 2014 (Back) TCCC CA

---

[64] George Barbee et al., "Joint Trauma System Clinical Practice Guideline: Chemical, Biological, Radiological and Nuclear (CBRN) Injury" (The Department of Defense Center of Excellence for Trauma, May 1, 2018), https://jts.health.mil/assets/docs/cpgs/Chemical_Biological,_Radiological_Nuclear_Injury_Part1_Initial_Response_01_May_2018_ID69.pdf.

Conclusion

As mentioned at the beginning of this book, the world is full of hazards. Individuals and communities expect their first responders, including fire, police, EMS, other disaster responders, and their medical system to both know what to do and to do it. First responders clear a tree which has fallen across a road or lift an elderly woman who has fallen in her hallway. They calm domestic tension and save victims in a major apartment fire. They find lost hikers, rescue stranded boaters, and mitigate chemical spills. Almost 2/3 of firefighters, and many other first responders, are volunteers. They protect their communities and receive little besides satisfaction for their efforts. Disaster relief workers often come later but still encounter dangerous hazards. Amidst this huge variety of tasks and workers, first responders need to know WMD/CBRN/HAZMAT.

Hazardous materials (HAZMAT) incidents are more common than most people realize, as almost every building and vehicle has a chemical toxin. Large HAZMAT calls, such as an overturned railroad car or tanker truck, occur infrequently. Calls involving weapons of mass destruction (WMD), whether chemical, biological, radiological, or nuclear (CBRN), are rarer still. Most first responders have never responded to a WMD/CBRN call and never will. Some may believe that it is pointless to prepare for WMD/CBRN events due to their rarity. A few may think that such events are so awful or so complicated that they can't do anything anyway. Some in small rural communities like ours might think that WMD/CBRN training is useful for big cities but not relevant to where we are.

WMD/CBRN agents have proliferated, as has the number and skill of actors who are capable of using them. Whether by accident or attack, the risk to our communities is growing daily. This book aims to train responders at all levels to manage that risk. The short outlines, summaries, tables, and figures contained herein, drawn from a recent lecture to Dr. Stagger's Medical Director's group in Southern West Virginia, are meant to quickly provide critical information for training, review, and response.

I hope that this book is especially useful for communities like ours, small and rural, with limited resources. As you think of items in this book that should be added, subtracted, better explained, or better presented, please let me know at the mdharrisinstitute@gmail.com.

References

Armed Forces Radiobiology Research Institute. "MEDICAL MANAGEMENT of RADIOLOGICAL CASUALTIES." Bethesda, MD: Military Medical Operations, July 2013. https://afrri.usuhs.edu/sites/default/files/2020-07/4edmmrchandbook.pdf.

Banks, Daniel E., ed. *Medical Management of Chemical Casualties Handbook*. 5th ed. Government Printing Office, 2014. https://medcoe.army.mil/borden-tb-med-mgmt-chemical-casualties.

Barbee, George, Devin DeFeo, Chris Gonzalez, Jill Harvilchuck, Carl Hoover, James Madsen, Joshua Perez, et al. "Joint Trauma System Clinical Practice Guideline: Chemical, Biological, Radiological and Nuclear (CBRN) Injury." The Department of Defense Center of Excellence for Trauma, May 1, 2018. https://jts.health.mil/assets/docs/cpgs/Chemical_Biological,_Radiological_Nuclear_Injury_Part1_Initial_Response_01_May_2018_ID69.pdf.

Bland, Steven A. "Chemical, Biological, Radiological and Nuclear (CBRN) Casualty Management Principles." *Conflict and Catastrophe Medicine*, November 22, 2013, 747–70. https://doi.org/10.1007/978-1-4471-2927-1_46.

Bureau of Labor Statstics, U.S. Department of Labor. *The Economics Daily*. "Fatal Chemical Inhalations in the Workplace up in 2017." *Bls.gov*, October 24, 2019. https://www.bls.gov/opub/ted/2019/fatal-chemical-inhalations-in-the-workplace-up-in-2017.htm.

Centers for Disease Control and Prevention. "Anthrax," 2020. https://www.cdc.gov/anthrax/.

Centers for Disease Control and Prevention. "Botulism," 2019. https://www.cdc.gov/botulism/.

Centers for Disease Control and Prevention. "CDC Radiation Emergencies | Facts about Prussian Blue," April 25, 2019. https://www.cdc.gov/nceh/radiation/emergencies/prussianblue.htm.

Centers for Disease Control and Prevention. "Chemicals by Category." www.cdc.gov, April 4, 2022. https://www.cdc.gov/chemicalemergencies/hcp/chemicals-by-category.html.

Centers for Disease Control and Prevention. "Decontamination for Yourself and Others," February 6, 2020. https://www.cdc.gov/nceh/multimedia/infographics/decontamination.html.

Centers for Disease Control and Prevention. "Dirty Bomb or Radiological Dispersal Device | Chemicals, Radiation and Toxicology Infographics | NCEH," February 6, 2020. https://www.cdc.gov/nceh/multimedia/infographics/dirty_bomb_radiological_dispersal_device.html.

Centers for Disease Control and Prevention. "How Potassium Iodide (KI) Works." n.d. https://www.cdc.gov/nceh/radiation/emergencies/pdf/infographic_ki.pdf.

Centers for Disease Control and Prevention. "Nuclear Power Plant Accidents | Chemicals, Radiation and Toxicology Infographics | NCEH." www.cdc.gov, February 6, 2020. https://www.cdc.gov/nceh/multimedia/infographics/nuclear_power_plant_accidents.html.

———. "Nuclear Weapon | Chemicals, Radiation and Toxicology Infographics | NCEH." Centers for Disease Control and Prevention, February 6, 2020. https://www.cdc.gov/nceh/multimedia/infographics/nuclear_weapon.html.

Centers for Disease Control and Prevention. "Plague," 2019. https://www.cdc.gov/plague/.

Centers for Disease Control and Prevention. "Radiation Contamination versus Exposure," March 25, 2022. https://www.cdc.gov/nceh/radiation/emergencies/pdf/infographic_contamination_versus_exposure.pdf.

Centers for disease Control and Prevention. "Signs & Symptoms ." Centers for Disease Control and Prevention, 2018. https://www.cdc.gov/hantavirus/hps/symptoms.html.

Centers for Disease Control and Prevention. "Smallpox," 2019. https://www.cdc.gov/smallpox/.

Centers for Disease Control and Preventioin. "Transportation Accidents | Chemicals, Radiation and Toxicology Infographics | NCEH." www.cdc.gov, January 23, 2023. https://www.cdc.gov/nceh/multimedia/infographics/transportation_accidents.html.

Centers for Disease Control and Prevention, "Tularemia," December 13, 2018, https://www.cdc.gov/tularemia/.

Centers for Disease Control and Prevention. "Where to Go in a Radiation Emergency | Chemicals, Radiation and Toxicology Infographics | NCEH," February 6, 2020. https://www.cdc.gov/nceh/multimedia/infographics/radiation_emergency.html.

Centers for Disease Control and Prevention. "Workplace Radiation Incidents | Chemicals, Radiation and Toxicology Infographics | NCEH." www.cdc.gov, January 23, 2023. https://www.cdc.gov/nceh/multimedia/infographics/workplace_radiation_incidents.html.

Cheshire, Harold T. "The Great Tartar Invasion of Europe." *The Slavonic Review* 5, no. 13 (1926): 89–105. https://www.jstor.org/stable/4202032.

CDC-Centers for Disease Control and Prevention. "CDC - Lice - Head Lice - General Information - Malathion FAQs." www.cdc.gov, September 17, 2020. https://www.cdc.gov/parasites/lice/head/gen_info/faqs_malathion.html.

Ciottone, Gregory R. *Disaster Medicine*. Philadelphia: Elsevier/Mosby, 2016.

Joint Trauma System Clinical Practice Guideline 1 and 2, https://jts.health.mil/index.cfm/PI_CPGs/cpgs.

International Association of Fire Chiefs, and National Fire Protection Association. *Fundamentals of Fire Fighter Skills and Hazardous Materials Response*. Burlington, MA: Jones & Bartlett Learning, 2020.

Little, Becky. "How Opioids Were Used as Weapons during the Moscow Theater Hostage Crisis." HISTORY, August 23, 2018. https://www.history.com/news/opioid-chemical-weapons-moscow-theater-hostage-crisis.

Pelley, Janet. "Number of Chemicals in Commerce Has Been Vastly Underestimated ." Acs.org. Chemical and Engineering News, American Chemical Society, February 12, 2020. https://cen.acs.org/policy/chemical-regulation/Number-chemicals-commerce-vastly-underestimated/98/i7.

Harris, Sheldon H. *Factories of Death : Japanese Biological Warfare 1932-45 and the American Cover-Up*. Routledge, 2015.

Shirer, William L. *The Rise and Fall of the Third Reich: A History of Nazi Germany*. 1960. Reprint, New York: Simon & Schuster, 2011.

Simons, Erica. "Faith, Fanaticism, and Fear: Aum Shinrikyo--the Birth and Death of a Terrorist Organization | Office of Justice Programs." www.ojp.gov, 2006. https://www.ojp.gov/ncjrs/virtual-library/abstracts/faith-fanaticism-and-fear-aum-shinrikyo-birth-and-death-terrorist.

Soloway, Rose Ann Gould. "Pesticide and Nerve Agents: Similar Poisons, Similar Symptoms." www.poison.org. Accessed August 2, 2023. https://www.poison.org/articles/pesticide-and-nerve-agent-commonality.

US EPA, Climate Change Division. "Nuclear Energy | a Student's Guide to Global Climate Change | US EPA." Epa.gov, May 9, 2017. https://archive.epa.gov/climatechange/kids/solutions/technologies/nuclear.html.

US EPA. "What Kinds of Consumer Products Contain Radioactive Materials?" US EPA, February 11, 2019. https://www.epa.gov/radiation/what-kinds-consumer-products-contain-radioactive-materials.

Wheelis, Mark. "Biological Warfare at the 1346 Siege of Caffa." *Emerging Infectious Diseases* 8, no. 9 (September 2002): 971–75. https://doi.org/10.3201/eid0809.010536.

www.ojp.gov. "4. Introduction to CB Decontaminants." OJP, n.d. Accessed August 2, 2023.

18 U.S. Code § 2332a - Use of weapons of mass destruction, https://www.law.cornell.edu/uscode/text/18/2332a.

Made in United States
Orlando, FL
07 November 2026

90337519R00039